Screams of Pleasure

Guide to Extraordinary Sex for those with Erectile Dysfunction

First Edition

Robert J. Rubel, PhD

Screams of Pleasure

Guide to Extraordinary Sex for those with Erectile Dysfunction

First Edition

Published by The Nazca Plains Corporation
Las Vegas, Nevada
2009

ISBN: 978-1-935509-00-4

Published by

The Nazca Plains Corporation ®
4640 Paradise Rd, Suite 141
Las Vegas, NV 89109-8000

Cover, Blake Stephens
Art Direction Blake Stephens

Foreword

Most men want to be good lovers. Most men want to please their female partners. Unfortunately, exactly how to please a female lover is a mystery to many men — and good instruction is very difficult to find.

By writing this book, Robert Rubel has done a very great deal to remedy that situation. Here, in this one volume, is absolutely first-rate information about the who, what, where, when, why, and how of creating an intensely pleasurable sexual experience for a woman.

The reader will learn about uniquely female anatomy and physiology, including what is and what is not involved in the controversial topic (and act) of "female ejaculation." The reader will further learn the whys and wherefores of using a wide variety of vibrators and dildos.

The extensive and detailed chapters on how to use one's hands and one's mouth on a female lover are some of the best material ever written on the subject. In a warm and friendly manner, he provides numerous techniques in highly usable detail, along with the proper attitude towards techniques in particular — and love-making in general. An entire chapter is devoted to the delicate erotic art of shaving a woman. There is even an excellent chapter on the rarely written topic of analingus. Safety and hygiene are covered completely and in specific detail throughout the book — while still preserving the loving and erotic mood of the material.

Everything is covered in loving detail, including the details of setting the scene, such as excellent tips on how to arrange the lighting and what music to use.

Robert is careful to approach his female lover as an entire human person. The book contains a very good chapter on negotiation and discussion of sexual matters, along with some very excellent advice on how a man can relate to his lover in a productive way outside the bedroom.

All in all, this book is a very useful and wonderful addition to the body of knowledge regarding how to make the sexual experience far more pleasurable for women. I suspect that Robert will be getting a fairly large number of letters of gratitude from women who have been lucky enough to receive the attentions of men who have used this book to educate themselves.

May the pleasure and satisfaction for all involved only increase!

Jay Wiseman
July 2, 2007
San Francisco, California

Author of:

SM101: A Realistic Introduction (Greenery, 1998)

Jay Wiseman's Erotic Bondage Handbook (Greenery, 2000)

Tricks To Please A Woman (Greenery, 2002)

The Toybag Guide to Dungeon Emergencies and Supplies (Greenery, 2004)

Tricks…To Please A Man (Greenery, 2004)

Jay's books and videos are available from a wide variety of vendors.
www.jaywiseman.com

Dedication

This book is dedicated to the many ladies who have helped to educate me over the years. Particularly, I am deeply thankful for having been shown…

- How to make an evening special through role play. She would come to the dinner table dressed in breathtakingly stunning fetish wear or lingerie — garter belt, hose, high heels. It brought out the best in me and filled our evenings with beauty and elegance. I've never had a hotter lover in my life.

- The importance of connection. How, with one lady in particular, we could stare into one another's eyes during sexual play and each find ourselves sucked into the other — and into another world. It was always eerie, because we usually submerged together. It was not an accident; it was an experience that she and I repeated often. Connection continues to be important with other sex partners, but this one lady was different, and dramatically so.

- The joy some women have in expressing their sexual passion for the pure fun of it, without any inhibitions. These women throw themselves into sex with their whole beings, and it strongly affects the quality of sexual play.

- That it's just as much fun being wrestled to the floor as it is to wrestle a lady to the floor. But what else is sex **play**?
- How to slow down in lovemaking, turning sexual evenings into hours of foreplay augmented by sensual scene-music playing in candle-lit and flower-scented rooms.
- That women, who previously never ejaculated (or even believed that it was possible), end up soaking towel after towel, to their utter amazement.
- That mastering the art of "stair-stepping" the woman's sexual arousal could consistently lead to ear-splitting orgasmic screams — even from ladies who later claimed a history of being non-verbal.
- That there is a huge difference between women who are okay with fellatio and those few who are remarkable at it, but that's the topic of another book.
- That some women who invite you over for an evening of sex want to start out with non-traditional activities such as spanking. Some women are willing to travel substantial distances so long as the sexual play is augmented with more adventurous play.
- That one can achieve incredible bonding and closeness with a partner on an intellectual/cerebral level without having much (or any) of the sexual component. From this lady, I learned that there are many Paths to the Answer.
- That all the skills in this book can be augmented when the lady you're playing with is also in love with you. Personally, I've never connected sex with love, but this lady does, and I'm surprised at how she plays differently with me than she plays with other partners.
- That all this can be done — that the lady can experience this wide range of pleasure — quite separate and apart from penile penetration.

Robert J. Rubel
Spring, 2009

Acknowledgements

When I completed the first draft, it was Karen Martin (an author in her own right) who performed the initial concept edit for flow, tone, voice, and meaning. She was able to redirect my focus so that subsequent drafts were much tighter.

Next, Jay Wiseman (author, attorney, and all-around good-guy) stands out for helping to shape this book to be what it is now. His close editing has been a true gift. Jay's sensitivity to sentence phrasing, his alertness to health and safety issues, and his lawyerly adroitness at steering me away from social/political missteps has repeatedly rescued me.

I am particularly indebted to Melinda for making four major detailed editorial passes at this work. Her work has made it much easier for me to write this book, while also making it much easier for you to read this book. Melinda also deserves recognition for being one of the key ladies to serve as a practice subject as I worked out many of this book's details. Also, I thank Melinda for often being my demo model when I make presentations on this topic around the country. She is very vocally responsive and adds a good bit to these presentations.

I particularly thank Katie Burgess, my illustrator. I know the assignment that I posted on Craigslist sounded a little unbelievable, and I thank you for having the guts to answer the ad. It's been a real treat to work with you.

Table of Contents

PART IV: LIGHT, CAMERA, ACTION

Part I

How to Navigate This Book

Chapter One

Important Basic Material

For most men, sex lies at the core of their relationship with women. Being blunt about it, a guy can have a great time having a beer with other guys without worrying about whether his drinking is okay, but when it's time for sexual play, that same man cares a great deal about how good a job he thinks he can do in bed. Unfortunately, his rating of his own sexual performance is likely to be quite different from his lady's rating of his performance, but that's beside the point. The point is, for many men, how well he can perform in bed affects his sexual self-image. His sexual self-image affects the way he relates to his lady. He'll notice if his lady isn't enthusiastic about making love with him. Many marriages ultimately end over the issue of sex.

In our culture, in Western culture, sexual performance mostly means intercourse. Penile play. So, when a guy can't get hard enough for intercourse, it can lead to a wide range of other problems/issues within his relationship. He may become withdrawn; he may take up hobbies and interests that become very time-consuming; he may start to withdraw emotionally from his partner. I know of a number of cases where the man simply has chosen to stop having intimate relations with his wife.

It doesn't have to be that way.

Men, there are many, many ways to bring pleasure and sexual playfulness into a relationship without the heavy emphasis on using your penis. In fact, once you start building upon —

and augmenting — what you already know about playing with a lady, I think that you'll be surprised with all the available options. This book is a playbook of sorts. This book offers extensive guidance and suggestions about how you can have hours of fun with a lady and re-establish your place in your own (and her) sexual world without relying on your penis.

As Dossie Easton and Janet Hardy say in the opening pages of their book Radical Ecstasy, this book is not exactly about *answers*, it's really about two other things: changing your approach to women, and exploring some new techniques for providing non-intercourse sexual pleasuring. It is the goal of this book to help propel you on your path to becoming an even greater lover than you are, today — or have ever been.

I certainly recognize that most men have their own preferred styles and techniques when it comes to sexual play. Some men are extremely inventive and experimental, and are tremendously successful at creating memorable sexual encounters. Other men seem to pay more attention to pleasing themselves than they do to pleasing the woman. Still other men may feel a bit lost in this arena, whether or not they admit it. I mention this, because I speak with a lot of ladies about their experiences with men. The report from the field, guys, is that the vast majority of men spend only a brief amount of time on foreplay, and are too anxious to get down to intercourse, anyway. I'm mentioning this at the outset because, from what I hear from the ladies, many of their sexual experiences with men start out as a huge yawn and spirals downward from there.

This book is specifically designed to change that. This book is specifically designed to provide an entire path of sexual play that is different from, but parallel to, sex play involving intercourse. If you're interested in taking my advice, this stuff comes first. And, for many men, may represent the majority of sexual play with a woman.

Your partner is very likely to take a renewed interest in you if you are able to master both the *techniques* and, perhaps more importantly, the *spirit* of this book. Don't worry, you'll get "pleased" in the end, but she's first. The more you give to her, the more time, care, and enthusiasm she will give back to you. It's as close to a guarantee as I can give as a writer: mastering this book will transform your life.

> "Too many men never use their hands to really explore their partners' bodies. They kiss and go right for her pants, perhaps with a short detour at her breasts. If you have participated in this kind of unbecoming behavior, leave it in the past! She wants her whole body to be touched and awakened, the nerve endings that extend along and beyond her whole spine to be ignited with touch." Lesbian Sex Secrets for Men, p. 122

In this book, I take two separate approaches with the single goal of broadening your sexual skills.

First, I'll focus on some of your own activities and behaviors that you may want to consider changing in order make the woman look forward to your sexual advances. These are the kinds of behaviors that tend to help to put a lady in a receptive mood for intimacy of any kind. Here, we're going for behaviors and attitudes that go beyond physical pleasure and cross over into the realm of relationship enhancement. Being a truly great lover involves your mind-set as much as it does your physical techniques. It is my opinion that to become a great lover, you must be in tune with the ways women process your actions — or lack of actions. For starters, this means:

- Being alert to her moods and gestures; her body language as well as what she is and is *not* saying
- Moving and touching at a pace much slower than you may now use — reveling in the experience of her body while letting her share yours
- Checking in with her constantly to ensure that what you are doing is, in fact, pleasurable for her

Being a great lover also means doing many little things around the house that will please her and make her feel loved. This is true whether you're bringing a new lady to your place, or if you've been with your partner for some time.

Foremost, your goal is to lessen both her unconscious emotional and sexual anxieties — and also your own. These tensions often restrict the ability of one or both partners to experience whole-body pleasure.

Second, I'll discuss and explain some forms of advanced sexual play, including chapters on:

- Oral sex
- The fine art of vibrator play
- Anal play, and
- Fingering techniques, from beginning to advanced.

Along the way, you'll learn how to combine most or all of your techniques in order to provide your lady with a spectacular sexual experience. Some of the sensations presented here — such as female ejaculation — may be new for her. Others — not so new, but set in a new context.

Because some men reading this book are still having intercourse, there are a few references to penile penetration; a few, but not many. This book is not intended to cover any sex positions or techniques that involve your penis — no vaginal intercourse, and no anal intercourse. There are plenty of outstanding books already in print that cover those areas.

Now, a quick word on gender, as it is used throughout this book. In the most general sense, I've written this book as though a man is playing with a woman. So *he* is playing with *her.* In real life, this book is gender-free. *She* may be directing *him,* or *she* may be playing with *her.* However, to avoid having to keep saying he/she — or any other clarifying combination of genders — please consider this book to be gender neutral and that gender references are being provided in the most commonly occurring fashion; a man is playing sexually with a woman.

What is this Book all About?

This is a book about *improving* or *changing* your sex practices, a subject that is largely taboo. Can you imagine a man casually mentioning to another man, "I can't get hard anymore and I really miss my sex life." That would suck the air right out of the room. What can anyone say? "Gosh, sorry to hear that. What about those Redskins?" Same response if a guy were to say to his drinking buddies, "You know, with my ED, I don't know how to please my wife, anymore; I wish I still knew what to do." You can just feel the other men edging away.

Anyway, what can someone say as a casual response without revealing too much personal information? For example, could you imagine someone saying, "You know, I felt the same way and I took this class…" Yeah, right.

So, these topics are not often discussed among men. From what I can learn from women about relations with their current or previous partners, sexual preferences and sexual performance are topics carefully avoided. So, how's a guy to learn that he's not so hot in bed? How's a guy to learn that he can please a woman spectacularly without relying on his penis?

It's a problem. Particularly it's a problem because without candid discussions with your partner, many men already think that they're good lovers and are therefore disinclined even to consider any path leading to improvement.

So, here we go, starting out with a book designed to help a guy get a glimpse about some alternatives to sex-as-usual. Some alternatives that, if your heart is in it, will transform your sexual life.

Conceptual Overview

> This is not a book of basics. This is not a book for couples that are satisfied with traditional sex practices.
>
> This is a book for those of you who are willing to take some personal risk to become a little more sexually experimental. This is a book for men and women who want to have a rollicking good time with their sex partner(s) without depending upon a penis.
>
> This is also a book written for women who want some way of explaining to the man/men in their lives how to have sex with them.
>
> This is also a book for men who may have developed erectile dysfunction (ED), and want to add new tricks to their lovemaking skills that don't involve penile penetration.

It is the purpose of this book to add oral, digital, and sex toy techniques to your established sex play in order to provide a richer and fuller sexual experience than your lady may now be enjoying. This book is aimed at providing you with specific techniques or ways of being that mesh with these various stages of sexual play.

- Physical and psychological preparation
- Erotic foreplay
- Staging the build-up process
- Mastering touching techniques
- Rhythmic stimulation
- Eliciting full orgasm (and often, female ejaculation)
- Resolution — aftercare

If you're fairly new to techniques of advanced sexual play — whether you are 21 or 71 — you probably have some reading to do to augment the material presented in this book; Appendix A gives you a starting point. This is a carefully constructed list of books and other resources that I found to be extremely helpful in my own quest. They deal with female anatomy, clitoral play, G-spot play, vibrator play, and so forth. Over the years, I have done my best to apply lessons from these books to my various sex partners. I suspect that these additional resources will help you to consider many additional variations beyond the examples provided in this book.

An admission: I began reading about female orgasms many years ago because I had a relationship with a woman who appeared to be non-orgasmic. I found this fact/phenomenon so challenging that I set out on a study/research path to help her. I did not succeed, much to our mutual frustration and sadness. Other factors in her life prevented her from having orgasms, including her prescription drugs. But, in the process of trying to learn to give her orgasms, I seemed to have picked up skills that are unusual enough, that many of my subsequent sex partners continue asking whether they can come back for more. So, I'm passing on what I have learned.

Some Background: Setting the Stage

This book describes the kind of sexual play that has taken me years to develop. And, I'm acutely aware that many men who purchase this book have also spent years developing erotic play styles with women — and that many women who read this book have well-honed ideas about what pleases them. That said, I have offered these techniques with a sense of humility and with the sincere wish that they bring new excitement and variety to your sexual life. My goal is that all readers come away with the feeling that they've learned some new and interesting tips, techniques, and strategies.

In an effort to keep your interest, and in an effort to keep this book light and chatty, I've sometimes interspersed my own opinions or comments along with the activity's description. I've even made a few attempts at humor. Most of the sexual play described in this book is designed to be strung together into *one single episode*. That is, chapters in this book are designed to flow together in a single sexual play session. Once you hit the chapter on vibrator play, these techniques will usually overlap your techniques for oral play, which will also involve fingering play, which will ultimately transition into your intercourse play, if that's still an option. It's likely to take you up to two hours to accomplish all this sexual play.

As this book is primarily focused on men with erectile dysfunction, I'll presume that if you're interested on intercourse positions and tips, you'll pick up some of the great books that are available. Again, this book is intended to help you create an evening of sex that can be independent of intercourse.

A Full-blown "Evening Event" May Look Something Like This...

- Setting the scene — lights, incense, candles, and music
- Candlelit dinner
- Erotic shaving
- Sensation play — touching her with feathers or other items that might not otherwise be touched to her skin — in order to create a pleasant, relaxed mood
- Oils and massage, hand and foot worship
- Vibrators (external and internal) and dildos

- Licking and fingering — cunnilingus combined with touching all the right spots
- Intercourse — if that is still an option

Much of this sexual play involves *technique,* as much as it involves a *sex toy.* Toys (such as vibrators or dildos) will only get you so far; their successful application depends upon learning how to play the woman like an instrument. To do this, you have to learn to read her reactions and then tailor your own actions accordingly. In the beginning, this involves interaction — doing something and then asking for feedback.

My goals are to help you put a wide range of skills and activities together that create magical sexual experiences, and to get you to consider re-trying some sex toys or techniques that may not have been successful the first time or two you tried them, or that you have used a time or two and then set aside for some reason or another.

Stair-stepping: Controlling the Sexual Play

Stair-stepping means that once you get the woman to a certain level of stimulation, you back off a little. Then you rebuild to a slightly higher level of stimulation, and then you back off a little. Then you build... This can go on for quite awhile — often more than an hour (with some breaks interspersed). At the end, after her ecstatic scream at orgasm, she may well burst into tears at the emotional release. You've just given her a cathartic experience.

Here are some tips for stair-stepping — the cycle that calls for you to build-up, back-off, and restart the build-up cycle over and over again. For the first two or three cycles, you're likely to be able simply to change your area of stimulation a little to get her to cool down a bit. But, as you build her higher and higher, you may wish to become a bit more playfully aggressive. For example, after perhaps three or four cycles, simply stop playing with her and take a break by starting a conversation or asking her if she'd like a chocolate-covered strawberry.

Because you've asked her to *think* rather than to *feel,* this will immediately snap her back into her head. Your statement is likely to illicit, "Huh? What? You're not serious! You can't stop now! No, come back." To which you reply lightly, "No, really, I know just the CD to put on (drink to get, snack to fix). Don't worry, this way we can just start over. By the way, while I'm up, would you like more wine?"

Of course, if your partner isn't a playful sort, this may kill your evening, so you have to use some judgment with this. The tricks you use to slow her down depend on each of your personalities.

Your skills in determining when to stop for a break and when to keep going will increase to the extent that you learn to observe your partner's reactions and feed off them. This includes her physical positions, her breathing, and the noises she makes. Your very serious job is to attend to her, to monitor her, and to listen to her. Oh yes, watch her hands, because how she moves and positions them can often help you determine how aroused she is.

Some Definitions

Because some of the material in this book wanders a little bit into the world of adventurous sex, I've provided some definitions to terms that should help you understand some of the concepts that I present.

If you run across any term you don't already know — or it seems that I may be hinting at something that you're not quite getting — try an Internet search.

Terms Relating to the Mental State

- ***Anchoring:*** Anchoring is a term from the world of hypnosis and neuro-linguistic programming (NLP). It refers to the process by which memory recall, state change, or other responses, become associated with (anchored to) some stimulus, in such a way that perception of the stimulus (the anchor) leads by reflex to the anchored response. As applied in this book, you can anchor various erotic responses to your lady during sexual play. For example, when she gets into a fully aroused state, pinch her earlobe a bit (not a lot). Once anchored (which could take a few repetitions), pinching her earlobe in the middle of the day can cause her to *change her state,* and to become sexually aroused. Those who practice NLP use anchoring to facilitate state management. (To learn a bit about how to do this, see: http://www.medzilla.com/firstimpressions.html)
- ***State:*** In everyday conversation, it's not unusual to describe someone as being in a "state" of some kind — a state of panic, a state of boredom, a state of bliss. Dictionaries tend to describe state as *the condition of a person.* In NLP, "state" has

a similar, but more specific meaning. There, it refers to the way a person presents him/herself at any moment in time, as a function of the mix of everything physical and mental going on with that person.

- ***State change:*** Something done by a person him/herself or something acting upon a person can change their *state*. As used in this book, *state change* refers to some action taken on the part of the man to change the woman's state from one level of arousal to another. The man may use subtle state change techniques to slightly raise or lower the lady's level of arousal in order to stair-step the overall sexual tension of the evening.

- ***Headspace:*** This term is sometimes used to describe someone deeply absorbed with an activity — often, so absorbed that outside sounds can disappear. This condition (that can be experienced by either partner) really speaks to the issue of *concentration* and *focus.*

Terms Related to Sexual Play

- ***Safe, Responsible, and Consensual:***

  - SAFE: While most people consider the physical act of sex to be safe, you need to be concerned with certain health issues when it comes to some of the techniques described in this book. For this reason, I've included safety warnings for you as you read through the various techniques.

  - RESPONSIBLE: If you are unsure about certain techniques, or want to try more advanced techniques found in adventuresome sex, you should seek specialized guidance from others who are skilled in these areas. This is an important part of playing responsibly.

  - CONSENSUAL: The sexual activity described in this book is for consenting adults, only. As I'm describing methods of turning your lovemaking into a very special (and possibly spiritual) experience, non-consensual sex clearly has no place in this process.

- ***Hard Limit:*** This term is applied to an activity that either partner considers an absolute, complete, total "No." For example, some ladies absolutely will not allow a man to put her toes in his mouth, or stick his tongue in her ear. Physical conditions also dictate hard limits. While she is perfectly happy to allow you to touch her all over in private, she is not likely to think it's very funny if you try that in church. Hard limit.

- ***Landmine:*** A person is said to have hit a landmine when one or the other partner inadvertently stumbles upon something that neither person had realized would be upsetting to the other partner. You'll know you've hit one if either partner's reaction to this event is extremely dramatic — way out of proportion to the event itself.

  Psychological landmines are far more common than physical landmines. You say something you think is completely innocuous and your partner becomes angry, or becomes physically aggressive, or bursts into tears. What was said triggered a memory of some prior experience(s) that neither of you could have known about. I've seen this happen *very vividly* with a man who had just started to have sex with his partner of about eight months. As we were all joking around, she made a comment using a somewhat coarse word to describe herself. That one word absolutely ended the night. Right then. No recovery possible. He told her to get dressed immediately, and that they were leaving. I was extremely upset about this, as I thought that I had done something to offend my guest. I had absolutely no clue what had just happened until I called him the next day. The word she had used that so upset him was not a hot-button for me, so I had a hard time even remembering that she had said it.

  In physical play, you may pull out a toy or start to touch/lick her in some place that seems perfectly normal to you, but that triggers a shocking reaction that surprises both of you. I once saw a demonstration where the instructor started to pick up a realistic-looking dildo to demonstrate a point on his volunteer demo-subject. Total landmine for her; her reaction was clearly apparent to all of us in the audience. Her body stiffened and there was a look of terror on her face. This immediately shut down the demonstration as the presenter now focused on working through the emotional trauma with the lady.

Terms Related to Play

- ***Toy:*** A sex toy is anything you or your partner selects to augment your own physical body during sex play. It can be something purchased (a vibrator) or something adapted from everyday life (a feather).

- ***Inside or Outside Vibrators:*** An inside vibrating sex toy is primarily designed to be inserted vaginally or anally, while an outside vibrator is primarily designed to be used on the surface of the skin. There is a certain amount of overlap, here.

Terms Related to Safety

- ***Fluid Bonded:*** Fluid bonding refers to the relationship between partners who are used to exchanging bodily fluids. Because they are fluid bonded, the couple no longer needs to practice safer sex with one another. Risky sex is defined as having unprotected sex with someone other than your usual partner. With almost all kinds of oral sex with a new partner, you'll not only put yourself at risk of catching an sexually transmitted infection (STI), but the next time you have sex with your usual partner, you will have put her at risk, too.

- ***Protection:*** Some barrier between you (or a toy that you are using) and the lady. This can be a condom on you or on a toy, or a glove on your hand. The general idea is that it is a physical barrier to transferring body fluids between sexual partners.

Chapter Summary

Some kinds of sexual activities with a partner can achieve unusual — even spiritual — dimensions. You don't need to use your penis to get there. When your intentions are aligned with your activities the results can be magical. To bring your partner to this level, it helps if you have a wide repertoire of skills and talents, a well-honed ability to read your lady's moods and sexual reactions, and the sensitivity to know what actions and techniques you need to change in order to keep her heading down the path that you have designed for her.

I've mentioned that at the end of a full sexual play session with your lady, she may start to cry from the cathartic emotional release, or she may actually have a lovely floating feeling for some time after you've stop playing. I also explained the meanings of a few words that may be new to you.

I explained that this book covers about everything under the sun except intercourse, which I leave to the many experts who have written competently about it. Everything covered here is designed to be used in a typical evening of sexual play I explained that this kind of sexual play involves *techniques* as much as it involves *toys*, and I introduced the idea of stair-stepping the evening's action in order to build to higher and higher levels of sexual stimulation with your lady. In that regard, I set out the stages of a typical sexual evening designed to be a truly gourmet event.

Chapter Two

The Mental Component

Your success with techniques in this book depends to a large degree upon your mastery of the material in this chapter. This book is unusual for a sex techniques book because of that very reason. The best techniques in the world are not very likely to succeed unless you have behaviors and a mind-set that enables the woman to relax enough to be able to accept your advanced skills. So, please consider this chapter to be of equal weight and importance to any of the techniques chapters.

The Physical Setting

What does your sexual play environment look like? What are you doing to make the physical area special/gorgeous? Once again, regularly repeating some of these next tips may serve to connect (anchor) the action with a sexual evening. If you can accomplish this, it will mean that as soon as she sees/smells/hears what you've done to make the environment special, she'll immediately begin to feel warm and slightly aroused. Said more formally, the change in the physical setting will cause an emotional state change and begin to put her in a mentally receptive mood for having a lovely evening — wherever it goes.

- ***Clutter:*** Are clothes left to be hung up? Are counter surfaces neat and clear of temporary items?

- ***Lights:*** Have you had dimmer controls put on your light switches? Have you taken steps — such as lowering the wattage of light bulbs — to make the room less bright and more romantic. (In my experience, few women enjoy playing sexually in brightly lit rooms.)

- ***Incense:*** Incense comes in a wide range of odors, from extremely sweet through a range of wood smells, to leather. Have you ever considered lighting some incense as a signal for the kind of evening you have in mind?

- ***Candles:*** Few things can improve the look of your dinner table better (and less expensively) than candles. They can go on coffee tables and mantles; they can go inside your fireplace in summertime, or even on the rim of many bathtubs.

- ***Flowers:*** You might consider not only buying flowers for your house on a weekly basis, but also arranging them for your partner. This is a little touch that goes a long way toward expressing your feelings to your partner. Also, it demonstrates that you, too, are working on the relationship.

- ***Music:*** Again, the kind of music that you select will add to or detract from the evening's mood. I encourage you to consider identifying some music that you only listen to when you're having a romantic/sexual evening. Make it special. One reason for doing this is that over time, that music becomes psychologically associated (anchored) with fabulous sex. Once that's done, you're likely to find that you both are in a much more sexual frame of mind when that music starts playing — even from the very first track.

- ***Dress:*** What are you wearing? Neat and tidy? A little dressy? How are you signaling to your lady that this is a special time? How can you say, "Let's get dressed up a little. Let's go out to dinner right here at home." It's easy to psychologically associate clothing with foreplay.

- ***Scent:*** Everything in the "anchoring" category certainly applies to your cologne, aftershave, or any additional scent you've applied. For example, I know of one man who applies a musk scent on nights he intends to play sexually. I know another man who has been experimenting with pheromones. In each of those cases, they chose not to apply any aftershave that could detract from their special scents. By the way, if your underarm deodorant has a scent, you might consider using something more neutral to avoid conflicting smells. In discussions with ladies, I've certainly heard any number of stories about how she met a man for an evening, but the first whiff of his cologne was so overpowering that she was immediately turned off. For many ladies, they've applied their own special scent; yours shouldn't overpower theirs. Not if you're trying to woo them.

- ***Set-up:*** Ever considered a "role play" scene?
  - You arrive home from work to find you've walked into the wrong house...
  - You're a repairman who, with your tool belt strapped around your waist (filled to overflowing with sex toys, of course), arrives for the "service call." The lady, not knowing that you'd put in a call for service, answers the door in a robe or negligee, having just stepped out of her bath, and says...
  - You decide to do the complete dinner setup yourself. You ask your partner to get especially dressed up for the evening. If she asks whether you're taking her out to dinner, be evasive. Keep her out of the kitchen and dining area until you, dressed also for the occasion, come in to get her from your bedroom, where she's been waiting for you. You seat her at table and you serve her.
  - Your lady has a high pressure job. In the morning, she told you she'd be home a little late. You decide to surprise her. You take the day off and hire a cleaning crew to come in for the day. You spend your time straightening up closets, the bedroom, dining room, kitchen area. As you're not a great cook, you conspire with one of your friends' wives to help you out with the dinner. When she walks in, the table is set with a centerpiece of flowers. You get the idea. "Right," you're saying. "Take time off of work to do this? You must live on another planet." Ok, so this is too extreme for you. I can accept that, though I don't think you should be too quick to dismiss it. Ultimately, the message is that you, too, have to work for the relationship, whatever form that work takes.

Sexual Play and the Five Senses

In order to give your lady the widest experience, you'll want to involve as many of her senses as you can. This section provides some examples of how to do this. The next section is intended to help you understand how to interpret which of your lady's five senses you need most to address.

Sight

Is your house/apartment/room clean? What is "clean"? When you walk into your own home with fresh eyes, is your reaction, "Oh, wow — what a neat place," or is it something of a catastrophe? To get a little distance from looking at your home through your own eyes, just imagine that you're bringing home a new lady for a sensual evening. Think how she would react if you had to say something like, "I'm sorry about the mess. Just close your eyes, Tasha; take my hand and I'll lead you to the bedroom... oops, sorry, I should have moved that box." Now look at your house again.

What have you done to show your woman that this is a special night for you?

- Do you have flowers arranged on the dining room table — and perhaps on the coffee table or bedside table?

- Did you buy her a little gift? Chocolate, perhaps?

- Have you pulled down the bed sheets? Sprayed the pillows with lavender? (Lavender is purported to have a calming effect. Anyway, by the time she recovers from the shock of all this, she'll probably be beyond calm. But you can probably revive her with the scent of roses.)

- Ever thought of buying a massage table? If so, now's the time to have it set up. Do you already have a little collection of vibrators and feathers? If so, are they already laid out... or are you going to risk breaking the romantic mood in order to open drawers and select items on the spur of the moment?

- If the weather is cold and you have a fireplace, is it preset and ready to light? How about candles — either placed inside the unlit fireplace or around the house?

- Are the lights dimmed? I think you'll find that muted light makes everyone and everything look better. Among other things, the amber glow will make you look a bit tanned. That's because the color temperature of dimmed lights is so much lower than bright white light, that it casts an orange glow.

Personal Note #1: The first thing I do when I move into a new house or apartment is to install dimmer switches in the living room, hallways, kitchen, master bedroom, master bathroom, and in any other important room. In my opinion, the last thing you want, when you bring your lady into your bedroom, is to have the lights on full intensity; what a mood-buster.

Sound

What do you know about choosing music to augment your sexual play? That is, have you selected music for the evening that is likely to augment or detract from the lady's experience of your time together? If you are classically inclined, how about a nocturne? If you enjoy New Age, how about "The Secret Door" by Mystic Ocean? Try asking her what she likes. There is actually a book out on the subject. Do an Internet search on: Sex Between the Beats. Appendix A lists a few CDs that I particularly like for this kind of sexual evening.

Tip #1: Use **two** stereo systems set up with **two** sets of speakers stacked one on top of the other. Play them at the same time. One system plays your romantic/sexual music; the other plays a 60-minute recording of a thunderstorm. The stereo system playing the thunderstorm can be an extremely modest used unit; you don't need quality sound to reproduce only the sound of rain and thunder. (The source for the storm-and-thunder CD is listed in Appendix A.)

Smell

Tried simmering cinnamon and brown sugar on the stove lately? Tried burning some piñon pine incense? Watch out with your choice of incense: many are too sickly sweet. Ever tried burning incense that smells like leather? How about daubing some musk scent on your chest before sex? We're going for masculine scents.

Have you ever used smudge sticks? These are bundles of sage or grasses used in various cleansing ceremonies by Native Americans. In my personal life, my lady — who is a healer — incorporates this into our pre-play ceremonies to create a sacred space for what is about to take place. This certainly signals to the woman that an evening with you is going to be unusual.

Taste

As you start out your evening together, consider a little food sharing. Sit face-to-face, naked or clothed, and feed her half a grape. Or a slice of banana, or a piece of chocolate brownie, or... (You might want to rent the 1963 movie *Tom Jones.* There is a food play scene in there that's worth the trouble of renting this DVD. It may help you better to understand the next paragraph.)

As with much of the material in this book, your own intention plays a key role. If you are feeding your partner half a grape, **how** you feed it to her is more important than the fact that you thought of doing so in the first place. You need to offer it to her as a seduction. Think for a minute: how did you end up with half a grape? Did you cut it in half? Or did you bite it in half slowly and languidly before slowly approaching her lips with the proffered item? Did you tease her with it or did you just say, “Oh, want a grape, Stephanie?”

Touch

Foot massage, anyone? Hand massage? Back rub?

Again, you're going for submersion, here. Your goal is to create a really special and relaxed evening that celebrates the ecstasy you feel, or intend to feel, as a result of being honored by being permitted to play sexually with this woman. If you expect her to consensually and erotically surrender her body to you; it's your job to make that erotic surrender a natural consequence of your forethought and behavior.

If you've managed the sights, sounds, smells, and tastes well to this point, the touches should lead to a spectacular evening that includes:

- Erotic shaving
- Whole body worship — feathers, massage, oils
- Vibrators

- Cunnilingus
- Fingering
- Intercourse — if that's an option

Processing Modalities

Now, after that detailed review of the use of the five senses in sexual play, let me take some time to discuss why working with the five senses is important for you. If you want more information on this next topic, try an Internet search for *processing modalities.*

People take in information in a number of ways. They also "process" information in certain ways. That is, if you're highly visual, you not only like things to look a certain way in your home, you may also actively search out lovely things to display in your home. If you have lots of wall decorations, this probably describes you. Related to the look of your house, if you're highly visual, you may pay a lot of attention to how you're dressed and how your lady is dressed. Personally, I really notice it when a lady takes the time to dress up a bit for our evening — hair, makeup, and clothing (particularly underclothing). These actions not only honor me, but they honor the special nature of our time together.

This being said, I realize that some people mainly connect with someone by touch, and are far less concerned about visual issues. This is relevant, because you're going to need to determine not only how *you* take in information, but also how your *lady* takes in information. If one person is high-visual and the other is high-kinesthetic, but neither of you know about differences in processing modalities, then the ways each of you communicate love or respect for the other may not coincide. That can be a problem. It can even be a problem that ends in break-up or divorce.

So, here's a quick review of the five categories of senses with some applications for your sexual (and relationship) life. As you see, they reflect the five senses and represent some of the different ways you may wish to adjust your normal preferences to meet her preferences, in order to help make her feel comfortable.

- ***Auditory:*** Purchase music in a genre that she particularly likes. Listen closely to how she phrases things, in order to learn how to speak to her with phrases that match the way she speaks. Any mismatch in speaking styles or in music choices are likely to set off alarm bells that she may not be able to name, but leave her with a slightly uncomfortable feeling.

- ***Visual:*** How you look, how the area looks, and how the toys look are critically important. You don't want to scare her or in any way make her uncomfortable. Remember, the more she has to *think,* the less she is simply *feeling.*

- ***Kinesthetic:*** Does she touch you? Does she specifically *not* touch you? How you touch her and where you touch her takes center stage. If one of you is strongly kinesthetic and one of you is strongly something else, you guys need to work this out. I know a couple where the woman would come up to her husband when he was working at his desk or reading a book, and touch him to communicate her love. The problem was, her husband was high visual and not at all kinesthetic. He told me that until he learned about these concepts, he would get furious at having his work concentration interrupted — and would stay upset for some time.

- ***Gustatory:*** For some ladies, you'll really please them by making (or taking them out to) a gourmet meal. For such women, you may want to involve some food play as foreplay. However, some women are the exact opposite. Not only do they not want to eat an elegant meal, but they would just as soon eat with their fingers. They prefer not to dine out. (Again, I'm not making this stuff up; I've lived it.)

- ***Olfactory:*** She may care a great deal about how you smell. In the first place, if she processes by smell, the greatest tip-off is that she probably sniffed your neck early in your relationship. You evidently passed that test, but now your cologne selection — and the smell of your home — become issues.

Sometimes, you don't have to speak to one another — sometimes the visual doesn't matter. Sometimes, it's just about your bodies. Never underestimate the power of teasing. Actually, teasing is much of what this book is about; teasing is foreplay.

Now, the generally accepted mythos is that men are visual, and women are auditory. That is, he wants to see the woman dressed seductively, and she wants to hear him say how sexy she looks. If some of these phrases don't come immediately to mind, please refer to Appendix B.

Note: after reading the appendix, please take some time to create some phrases that you, personally, could use with your particular partner. Major caution: These phrases must be honest and come from your being. Otherwise, they will sound like just another line and she'll lose interest immediately. Women have refined BS-detectors; you may find yourself in a non-recoverable situation if she suspects that you're manipulating her with sweet phrases.

Other Areas to Be Considered

Adaptability

Individual women are so different that your approach has to have wide breadth. On a practical level, none of the women with whom I have been intimate enjoyed exactly the same types of vibrators or the same sequencing. This probably surprised me far more than it will surprise you. You'll have to create a new sexual language for each woman with whom you play sexually. That means that you have to "speak woman." You're going to have to learn your lady by asking lots of questions and then, based upon what she tells you, practice ways of pleasing her. But the flip side of this is that your partner has to know her body and communicate her wants and needs. It seems as though few ladies are used to coaching a man (for fear of threatening his ego); similarly, it seems as though few men ask for coaching from their partner (because without feedback, men mostly think they're doing sex just fine).

Her Fears and Anxieties

Much of the material in this book has been designed to set up an environment and a series of activities calculated to take the lady's mind off of herself. Everybody brings a certain amount of baggage into a relationship, be it a one-night stand, a previous long-term relationship, or your current relationship. However, the sexual response of women — much more so than that of men — is connected to other kinds of thoughts. She is likely to start out worrying and fretting and brooding about some of the concerns that are listed below. These concerns, and others that are unique to your lady, have an impact upon how your evenings together turn out. To the extent that you are aware of — and sensitive to — these kinds of concerns, you will be able to substantially improve those evenings.

Examples of what ladies fret about...

- She will be concerned about how she thinks she looks to you in the clothes she chose for the evening, how she's fixed her hair, and the care she took to have her nails done. Unless you recognize this and acknowledge her for the time/care she has taken, you'll lose points. Lots of them. Learn to compliment your lady.
- She will be particularly sensitive to whether you'll like (or even notice) the lingerie she so carefully selected for the evening. (This can run into a lot of money; she may have purchased her lingerie just for your evening together.)
- Even if your relationship is established, the lady may have some lingering questions about whether you think her private parts look and/or taste good to you.
- If this is a new partner, she is very likely to be anxious about whether she can/will please you.
- Often, the lady will not be sure whether she can give herself permission to have sex with you. This is extremely relevant if the woman is recently out of a long-term marriage or relationship that she didn't end. It's also true if you have a long history of not being very sexually caring or attentive to your partner and she really doesn't want to have sex with you. Question: Just how nice have you been to your partner on an ongoing basis?
- Again, for new partners — the woman may be concerned about whether she can control you; she may fear being overwhelmed by your assertiveness. Also, she may have had bad prior sexual experiences that make her anxious in intimate situations. See Appendix A for more information.

As you can see, you may have quite a bit to overcome. That's why you're going to want to be particularly attentive in this chapter, for I will be suggesting ways to approach your lady that may be very different from your past behaviors.

As previously mentioned, much of the sexual play described here is aimed at helping you learn how to play your lady as though playing a particularly valuable instrument. Think about playing a piano for a moment — even if you don't really play a piano. Sometimes, the piano fingering (or playing with your lady) is very slow and light/delicate (lento, legato, or delicato); sometimes it's very hard, fast and enthusiastic (con forza, rapido, con fuoco).

Sometimes it's pretty much in one place; sometimes it covers all eight octaves, sometimes only two octaves. Regardless of where on the keyboard you are playing, the purpose is to create a lovely sound — and it's the sound that this instrument makes (be it piano or woman) that enables you to know whether or not you've mastered the art form. As a side note, many women make fairly consistent sounds when certain things are done to them, or when they are touched in certain ways. Thus, I am being quite literal when I say that when you are playing with your lady, you are, in fact "playing an instrument."

Mastering the material in this book is rather like mastering a new art form. When you're playing with a woman, whether a new partner, or an established partner, your goal is to discover what combination of your actions will result in her vibrating, moaning, squirming, screaming, and squirting.

The Context of Your Sexual Play

Among other things, pleasing a woman starts with:

- The way you're dressed when your lady shows up at your door — or you show up at her door ("showing up at the door" can certainly mean "when your wife gets home")
- How you act when you first see her — even if it's your wife coming out of the bathroom having just dressed for the occasion
- How you smile and what you say in the first two seconds that you see her (Yup, two seconds. She's timing you. It's a test. If you've been married 20 years, it's still a test. If you don't believe me, give her three drinks and ask her outright.)
- How you've set up the environment (music, lights, candles, incense)
- Whether your fingernails are clean (and manicured; a *sports manicure*, guys)
- Whether she likes the smell of your deodorant and aftershave

This starting list also includes her mental review of:

- What you have done for her lately
- The last time you brought flowers or candy or…

- The last time you took her out for dinner...
- How pleasing your general day-in-and-day-out demeanor/behavior is

> **Tip #2:** You must dress to attract the kind of woman you seek. If you're in an established relationship, how do you behave to make the evening sex play seem different from the way you've been all day long?

Ideas for dressing:

- You should wear clothing that your wife/SO/girlfriend found attractive at some point in your relationship. That can range from jeans to a tuxedo. In the middle, you might try lightly starched khakis and a sharp shirt. Remember the goal. You're trying to communicate to the lady that you've done a lot to make this evening special. Looking particularly sharp helps to deliver that message.
- Fashionable shirt? You might consider offering your lady an opportunity to take you to a mall and dress you as she would like to see you. Anyway, one of the fastest ways to a woman's heart is to say something like: "Honey, I know you love shopping at the mall. Why don't we zip down there and you can select a special shirt that you'd like to see me wear tonight. Then, we'll go shopping for some shoes for you for tonight. And — say what! — how about if we go out for lunch before we come home?" (Again, please refer to Appendix B for a list of similar expressions that may well transform your relationship with your partner.)
- You might consider making it a habit of always slightly overdressing, particularly when going out on a date — especially if the date is with your wife. Ladies always notice when you've clearly gone out of your way to dress up to honor them.
- Shoes shined? Even if your lady isn't into anything extravagant, she is very likely to appreciate nicely shined shoes. This is particularly true if you're in an established relationship. Shining your shoes before you get together will demonstrate to your lady your commitment to your relationship, as well as signal to her that the evening is special.

- How about your underwear? Are you wearing something really traditional, or something really sexy? Tried any interesting briefs, lately? The Internet is full of sites offering an extremely wide range of options. When was the last time you slipped off your trousers and the lady said, "Oh, those are *nice,* please turn around for me. Wow!" (I'm not making this up, I promise.)
- Belt reasonably new? Reasonably in-vogue? Dressy?

> **Tip #3:** Consider bringing some fantasy into this sensual play we're about to describe. Consider dressing your lady in a corset, hose, and heels. Consider starting out in a suit and tie or in nightclub wear. When I present at conventions, people often say, "We never dress up! We wouldn't feel comfortable." Okay, I still recommend that you figure out ways to help to make this kind of evening special, but this is in no way a requirement. That's why it's listed here as a tip.

Consider your physical condition. Are you fit and trim? Are you pretty much in the same shape as the woman you are seeking? Are you modeling the kind of body you wish your partner to have? If you were a hot woman, would you want to go to bed with someone whose body looks like yours?

If you're in an established relationship, do you actively help your partner...

- Take out the garbage?
- Do the dishes?
- Mop the floor?
- Vacuum the house?
- Chauffeur your kids around?
- Help with the grocery shopping?
- Take clothes to the cleaners?
- Ensure she has some free time to explore her own desires?

Do you…

- Pick up your clothing?
- Fold your own socks and underwear? (Another lifted eyebrow on that one?)
- Pick up *her* clothing? (I know. That one just threw you overboard.)

On the evening you intend to make love, did you…

- Set a beautiful candlelit dinner table for her?
- Ensure that the lighting was subdued and that your specially selected mood music was playing?
- Pay her compliments that you truly felt?

Said differently, what — exactly — are you doing to put the woman in the mood to be played with? What are you doing that makes this particular woman feel loved, cherished, and powerful? To get a better feel for this, consider yourself to be the woman and think how you would want to be treated if the evening is going to be one of sex play. This is particularly true if you're married where boredom and repetition so often set in. It's so traditional for the woman to do all the house-prep for dinner and such, just think what an impression you will make if you take all that over from time to time. Let her take a bubble bath while you do the running around. (At the risk of going too far, again, consider getting a small tray and — when she's in the bubble bath — bring her a nice drink with a single rose on that tray. Next time, she can treat you that way. You're leading by example, here.)

This brings us back to the previous question: Why are you playing with this woman? What are you trying to accomplish when you actually have a woman on your hands? Are you just trying to please yourself, or are you *Reveling in Woman*? I'm always humbled and amazed that I have a lady before me, naked and willing, who has invited me into this aspect of her life. I revel in the trust that she has placed in me. I'm reminded of the Bryan Adams song, "Have You Ever Really Loved a Woman?"

There are some early pitfalls in this game. Sometimes women don't know what pleases them. In many cases, they don't know their own bodies. They've never explored themselves and can't exactly tell you what they like or dislike. In other cases, they're not very in touch with their sexuality, particularly if post menopausal. It can be hard to determine exactly why she's appearing a bit stand-offish. This is where *technique* comes in. You're going to have to develop speaking, listening, and behavioral skills that will even let such a lady play sexually with you. Once playing, not only are you going to have to master the art of inquiry-and-feedback, but you also will have to know what each of your toys can offer the lady. If you are not used to behaving this way right now, it will take some practice.

As I keep mentioning, few women will tell you when you're not quite getting it right. She is unlikely to say anything, because every man wants to think he's a great lover, and women, wise as they are (and frequently culturally trained to want to please and nurture their man), won't rush in to burst that bubble or hurt your feelings. In such cases, your partner simply won't be very encouraging about being with you again.

By the way, this works both ways. You've undoubtedly encountered women who are so trained to traditional sex practices that they are simply not willing to stretch their limits. After a little probing, you're likely to conclude that this woman is not a candidate for new experiences. Although fine for her, this condition may lead to you to want to look elsewhere for more interesting sexual experiences.

As you've no doubt already discovered, each woman "drives" differently. Here's a parallel: While all cars have four wheels and an engine, pick a domestic car manufacturer and think of yourself driving through an obstacle course behind the wheels of a compact model, a full-sized model, and an SUV. While they're all operating pretty similarly, they won't feel the same. And they won't feel the same going around a tight turn at 65 mph. And they'll all go from 0-60 in very different times. Same with women.

That, then, brings us to a question: If each woman drives differently, how do you figure out how to drive the lady you're now playing with? Now, that's the question, isn't it.

And the answer is... communication is the key.

- Please keep in mind that women have a wide range of responses, from being non-orgasmic to being able to orgasm on command. What works great for one woman may not work very well (or at all) for another woman.

- As you're going along, ask her, "Which feels better, this or that..."

- While you don't want to break the mood of the evening, I strongly recommend that the next day you do a recap. Ask her what she liked and wishes more of, or didn't really like and wishes less of.

> **Tip #4:** When you're playing with her, and she's just had an ear-splitting orgasm, consider asking, "Does this mean you will come back?" You'll likely get a sexy chuckle out of her. This is even more relevant (and more appreciated) if you say this to your long-term partner/wife.

Negotiating Your Sexual Play

I know, you want to get to *the good stuff.* Well, as I keep saying, *the good stuff* won't be a lot of help unless you have built the proper foundations. Please hang in here, with me. All this matters in the end. Also, for those of you reading this book who have been with your partner for years and years, it's actually fairly likely you've never directly engaged these questions with her. You've derived your answers without ever verifying them. Imagine how flattered she'd now be to be asked some basic questions. (Oh, and has she ever asked *you* what she can do to please you? It's a two-way street, right?)

About Determining Her Likes and Dislikes

By discussing what your lady may like to do during your time together, you may be able to provide more variety in the sex play than you had previously considered. Similarly, failure to discuss your options before your evening of sex will limit what you will offer the lady.

Pre-sex negotiations can take unusual turns. For example, if you're a committed vibrator guy, you might bring out an array of vibrators to discuss with her. If you have other strong preferences (dare I say fetishes) this is a time to discuss them. You'll never know when you'll stumble upon someone else who has your particular preferences — or someone with nearly opposite sexual preferences.

One time, when I was negotiating sexual play with my partner for the evening, she commented that she really didn't like vibrators. And she wasn't very interested in receiving oral sex, and wasn't thrilled at fingering. Well, since those just about define my sexual foreplay, I was a little nonplussed. I couldn't see how this encounter was going to be very interesting for either of us. Said differently, while it was going to be fun to have intercourse with a new lady, she was not going to get from me the full range of sensual experiences that I could offer, and I was not going to be able to make this a special time for her.

- Ask if there is any part of her body that she would prefer that you not touch.
  - Stroking her face?
  - Touching or licking behind her ears?
  - Touching or gentle licking inside her ears?
  - Gently pinching, slapping, flicking, or biting her nipples?
  - Playing around her feet/toes?
- Once you've been with a lady a number of times, you may want to ask her whether you may be a little experimental with your licking. For example, if you'd really like to lick her armpits, she needs to know this in order to remove her deodorant. At this point, you will have to be specific in describing your proposed licking points, as some of these (such as here bellybutton) may be hard limits; if you're not specific during negotiations, you may hit a landmine and ruin your romantic evening. (Caution: If you try having this discussion with a brand new lady in pre-sex negotiations, she may be put off and think you're too weird for her.)
- Many people — both men and women — have secret fantasies about being spanked. Often, these are kept well-hidden. However, at some point in your relationship, you might want to probe this a little. You might ask whether she would enjoy a light spanking interspersed with the evening's sexual play. Here are some other topic ideas:
  - Hey, if you don't behave yourself, I'll have to bring a paddle, next time!
  - If you keep wiggling around like that, I may have to tie you up!
  - You know, I saw a book the other day on spanking (or some other sexual topic), would you like me to buy it so we can go through it together?

- Ask whether she has ever considered anal play.
    - Licking
    - Light touching
    - Slight penetration
    - Full anal penetration — dildo or penis

Once you initiate sexual play, be sure to check in frequently. Consider asking:

- Is this hard enough/too hard?
- Do you like me to touch more on the left or on the right?
- How about this vibrating frequency?
- How do you feel about anal vibes? Willing to try one?

About Foreplay and Penetration

Much as men want to penetrate women's bodies, women want to penetrate the psyche of the person living in the body they are playing with. Often, for a woman, the sexual experience is broadened through connection with the mind inside the man's body.

According to many women, guys usually have the idea that you start with a kiss, spend the minimum acceptable time playing with her breasts and genitals, and move right in for penetration. There are two problems with this. First, this way of thinking is neglecting the psychological and emotional parts of sex. These are the parts that involve communication and touching that are not goal-oriented. Second, you and your sex partner risk missing most of the fun of lingering and being with one another in an intimate setting. Additionally, it is not very likely that you will experience sexual magic during such an encounter. Sexual magic takes planning, focus, and concentration.

In this light, you might want to have a heart-to-heart discussion of what *she* wants out of the encounter and what *you* want out of it.

The Psychological Component

Why is this woman having sex with you? What's in it for *her?* Have you asked her? Is this your wife and she sort-of has to have sex with you? Is this lady spending the evening with you primarily because she hasn't been laid in a while, or is it that she is hoping for some kind of connection with you that is somehow different? If different, just how different — and what does *different* mean to her? Do you have a particular skill set that she might be seeking? Do you offer a particular form of fantasy fulfillment? Are you offering some form of taboo with your play? Does she seek role play or power exchange?

The bottom line is that it's important that your partner becomes aroused and excited. But, "aroused and excited" comes in all the colors of the rainbow. I urge you to work very hard to match your own foreplay techniques with your partner's foreplay wishes — even if they aren't exactly your foreplay wishes. In relationships, each side compromises on many subjects. She may try to negotiate with you about household chores; you may try to negotiate with her on where to go on vacations. Similarly, sexual foreplay may involve some give-and-take on each of your parts. However, if you want this woman to come back and play with you sexually on other occasions, you can be assured that if she says that she really likes to receive XYZ stimulation as warm-up, you're well-advised to learn how to do XYZ. When you hear, feel, and know that your partner is turned on, you can relax and get into the moment. Once you know that the woman has been pleasured with her kind of sex play, it's going to be easier to be uninhibited with your own kind of sex play. Now, there's less room for insecurity on both your parts — and more room to relax into the intimate/connected part of sex.

Pulling This All Together Before We Get to the Techniques

Determining Her Comfort Level

If you're playing with connection, if you're playing with the intention of making your partner fly, then you are going to have to be monitoring your partner very closely throughout the evening. In addition to monitoring her sounds very closely, you will have to monitor her breathing, the rigidity/tenseness of her body, her facial and vulva colors, and her hand motions. Hand motions are crucial; for many women, they are often the most visible sign of her state of sexual arousal. And by the way, you're likely to discover that as you're stimulating the woman, she may well want your physical touch; she wants one of your hands interlaced with hers. And other times, she wants just the opposite — she wants to be blindfolded and to feel as little of your body contact as possible while her personal fantasy plays out to the touch of your fingers, your vibrators, or your thrusting penis.

Staging

If you're going to get your partner to fly, you're going to have to master the art of staging or stair-stepping your sexual activity. However you are stimulating her, your sexual play has to build and fall back, build higher and fall back, build higher yet and fall back. Take your time. A full-blown cunnilingus/fingering/vibrator scene may take an hour or two. But what's the hurry? Once you've figured out how to do it, you're likely to go through many build-up-and-back-off cycles as the evening progresses. And if I don't miss my mark, you'll find that these are fabulous evenings for both of you.

Setting the Scene

The way you set up the environment leading to sexual play with your partner depends upon a few things, such as:

- Your own imagination
- Your budget
- How well you know your partner
- How much time/trouble/research you've spent before-hand determining what your partner thinks a hot romantic scene would look like/feel like/sound like
- The extent to which you buy into the material in this book and actually make it your own
- The willingness both of your lady and yourself to stretch your sexual boundaries

But this is all good stuff, and you should have lots of fun trying it out.

Chapter Summary

In many ways, this chapter holds the key to your successful application of all the tips and techniques described in this book. I began by discussing some fundamental details, such as how you've physically set up your home/apartment and your play space. I then provided a detailed discussion of ways of playing with her five senses. Not only the "how" of this stage, but also the "why" of it. Closely allied to this discussion, the next section reviewed processing modalities in order to help you understand the practical importance of the five senses. Next, I reviewed some about a lady's possible fears and anxieties, and ways you may help to calm those fears. All this was followed by a long list of specific activities that would affect the context of your sexual play, as well as the physical, psychological, and emotional components.

The next major section of this long chapter discussed the importance of negotiating the elements of this kind of sexual play. Many of the activities I've described in this book are likely to be new to her. For the sake of your future sexual play with the lady, it's wise to do some pre-play negotiating. From here, I went into more detail about the psychological and emotional components of sexual play, ending up with a serious discussion about the importance of closely monitoring your lady in order to determine whether or not you're continuing to bring her to even higher levels of arousal, or whether you're losing her.

Part II

About Her Body

Chapter Three

The Sexual Anatomy of Women

I know. You know all this stuff. Or do you?

Ladies tell me that very few men are really familiar with the specific parts of a woman's genitals. They go on to admit that they believe that few women are really familiar with their own private parts. My questions to perhaps 20 ladies about such areas as the A-spot, Skene's glands, and the size and shape of their cervix usually draw a blank stare. To ensure you and I all referring to the same anatomical parts, this section is presented as a quick review — but only about those parts that will most concern you in sexual play. This is certainly not intended as an anatomy lesson.

This chapter is divided into two sections: an overview of the territory, and then a specific discussion of erogenous hot spots.

Overview of Female Genitalia

Vulva

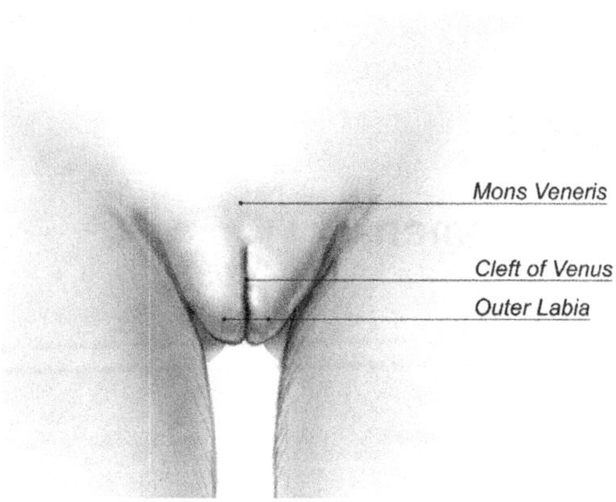

The external female genitals are collectively referred to as the vulva. All of the words below are part of the vulva. This is the area often referred to as the pussy, the cunt, or (confusingly incorrect), the vagina.

While some women will be turned on by the use of slang terms for body parts or sexual activities, many will be turned off. I've stripped almost all slang terms from this book. That said, if you do a search for "cunt" on Wikipedia and go down to the "usage" sections, you'd be entertained reading about its use over time and in various countries. I had not been aware that in a number of situations, the term is used to refer to men. For example, they point out that in England, this word is often used as a form of endearment when applied to men. News to me...

Mons Pubis or Mons Veneris

In females, the mons pubis is sometimes called the mons veneris (Latin, mound of Venus). It is the soft mound of flesh present just above the genitals, raised above the surrounding area due to a pad of fat lying just beneath it that protects the pubic bone. The mons veneris divides into the labia majora (literally "major lips") on either side of the furrow, known informally as the Cleft of Venus, and known medically as, the pudendal cleft. The inner lips contain the vaginal opening and other structures of the vulva. The fatty tissue of the mons veneris is sensitive to estrogen, causing a distinct mound to form with the onset of puberty.

Tip #5: Placing the flat of your palm on the *mons* just above the vulva and pressing down firmly while engaged in other genital play intensifies sensual feelings in some women. If it works that way for your lady, it should heighten her sensitivity to touch throughout her vulva.

Labia Majora

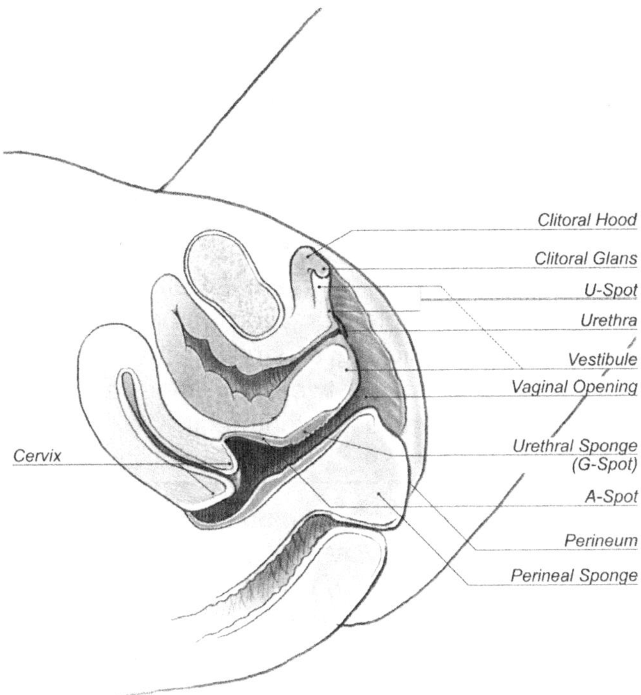

The outer lips of the vulva are called the labia majora. These are pads of fatty tissue that surround the vulva from the mons to the perineum. Unless the woman shaves, or is waxed, or has had laser treatment, the labia are covered with pubic hair. Whether or not shaved, this area contains numerous sweat and oil glands. As this entire area is sensitive to touch, you are likely to find that ladies like to be licked at the juncture of their crotch and their outer lips.

In adventurous sexual play, there are actually a wide range of activities that involve the vulva. If you're curious about this kind of play, I highly recommend that you purchase Jay Wiseman's SM-101: a Realistic Introduction (www.jaywiseman.com — full citation is found in Appendix A).

Personal Note #2: I find that many, many women appreciate some kinds of adventurous play — and often ask that it be interspersed with the activities described in this book.

Personal Note #3: While this may be counter-intuitive, you're likely to find that many women enjoy it if you carefully set your teeth around one of the outer lips, get a good grip, and back out. You'd be surprised how much *pulling* the outer lips can take. You'll want to get as much of that outer lip in your mouth as you can.

Labia Minora

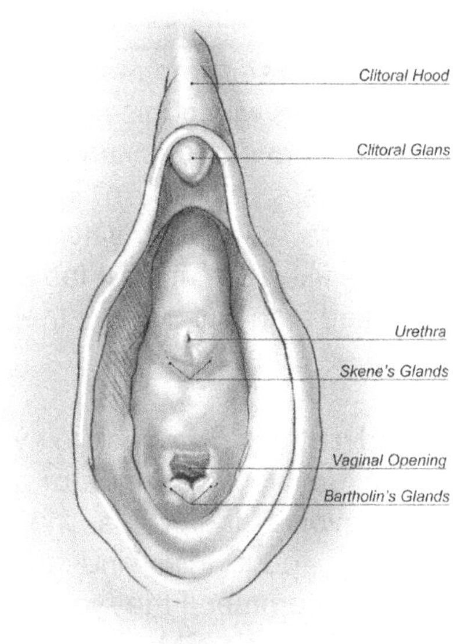

The labia minora — inner lips — are thin, fleshy tissues enclosed within the labia majora — outer lips. Their appearance varies widely between women, running the gamut from tiny lips that are hard to locate, to large lips that extend well beyond the outer lips. As both the inner and outer labia are extremely sensitive to touch and pressure, you may want to spend more time licking or stroking the outside of the inner lips (between the inner and outer lips) than has been your habit.

Tip #6: As a woman becomes more sexually excited, the inner lips may swell with blood. In some ladies, this can be quite pronounced; that influx of blood will cause the lips to darken. Because this is an involuntary indication of arousal, you should be monitoring both color and fleshiness of her inner lips.

Vagina

The vagina connects the vulva (outside the body) to the cervix of the uterus (inside the body). Although there is wide anatomical variation, a current British research project reported that the average vaginal canal ranges in size from 2.56" to 12.92" (Lloyd, Jillian et al *Female genital appearance: 'normality' unfolds,* BJOG: an International Journal of Obstetrics and Gynecology, May 2005, Vol. 112, pp. 643–646). Upon arousal, the vaginal canal elongates a certain amount to accommodate a penis or a sex toy. But, there is a limit to this elongation, and if you hit the back wall of the vagina with your penis, or with a sex toy, your lady is likely to let you know that you're hurting her.

While penis size is not correlated to a man's height or weight, vaginas tend to mirror body type. According to a 1996 British research study, bigger, taller women tend to have a somewhat longer vaginal canal. They also noted that age and child-bearing affect vaginal dimensions. The older you get, or the more kids you have, the bigger you become.

Tip #7: For many women, vaginal nerve endings are concentrated at the opening of the vaginal canal, not inside the canal. This is why playing around the vaginal opening is often more pleasurable for some women (softly fingering the opening and only putting your fingers in an inch or so when starting sexual play) than starting out with any kind of full insertion (fingers or penis). Many women report that once fingers or a penis is inside them, they mostly feel pressure.

Urethral Sponge

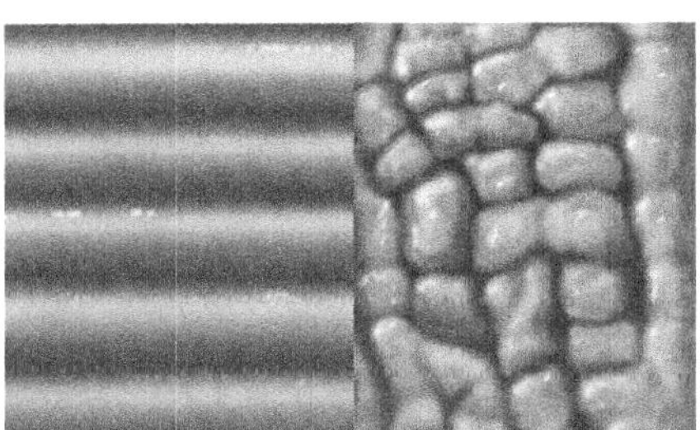

Smooth Tissue Spongy Tissue

According to Wikipedia, the urethral sponge is composed of erectile tissue that — during arousal — becomes swollen with blood, thus compressing the urethra. This action by the urethral sponge (with help from the pubococcygeus muscle) helps to prevent urination during sexual activity. The urethral sponge is often referred to simply as "spongy tissue."

The urethral sponge encompasses a large number of nerve endings, and can, therefore, be stimulated through the front wall of the vagina. Some women enjoy the rear-entry position of sexual intercourse (or dildos) for this reason, because the penis is often angled slightly downward and can stimulate the front wall of the vagina, and in turn, the urethral sponge. If you're using a dildo, this is what you're aiming for.

The urethral sponge is sometimes referred to generally as the G-spot (Gräfenberg spot), although some say that the two are separate. Some women experience intense pleasure from stimulation of the urethral sponge; others find the sensation neutral or even irritating. The urethral sponge also surrounds the clitoral nerve, and since the two are so closely interconnected, stimulation of the clitoris may stimulate the nerve endings of the urethral sponge. (See discussion of the G-spot, below.)

Perineum

The perineum is the short stretch of skin starting at the bottom of the vulva and extending to the anus. Another way of describing it is: the area that is neither part of the genitals nor part of the anus, but the region of skin between the two. This area is lined with nerve endings that are extremely sensitive to touch by finger or tongue. This area is known by a variety of slang expressions, depending on where in the English-speaking world you live. It is variously called the durf, guiche, grundle, chode, taint/t'ain't ('taint the anus or the vagina), or chad.

> **Tip #8:** You may wish to take a break from licking or fingering and lightly stroke that area. Remember, if you're stair-stepping your lady's arousal, you'll need some tricks to slow her down without bringing her totally out of her headspace of arousal and excitement.

Posterior or Perineal Sponge

I have a problem with this one. Not only are these terms rarely noted among sex tips, but I couldn't find any Internet sources that linked these terms to sexual activity. The Wikipedia definition of perineal sponge is: "A dense network of blood vessels that lies underneath the perineum." However, this definition is found in their description of the extensive parts of the *clitoris*, and not as a zone of sexual arousal. Worse, some of the anecdotal sex tip writers on Internet sites place this area below the vaginal opening (woman on back) while others claim that "perineal sponge" is synonymous with the *urethral sponge* and that it includes the G-spot. Clearly, you can't have it both ways.

Trying to make sense out of these two paragraphs, I conclude that the perineal sponge is covered by the area of skin that is medically known as the perineum. If you stroke it from the *inside* of the vagina, it feels good. If I'm wrong, here, healthcare professionals reading this section are encouraged to email me with the correct information; I'll include it in the next edition.

At any rate, the area I'm trying to discuss is a pad of erectile tissue — often felt as very smooth skin — located inside the vagina on the posterior vaginal wall. You can feel it when your lady is on her back and you insert one or two fingers downward, pointing toward her anus.

I think you're likely to get a good review from your lady if you alternate your inserted fingers between "pointing upward" and "pointing downward" positions. Try rotating between these two positions either slowly or quite rapidly, depending upon her state of arousal. As you repeatedly switch from the lower to the upper position, your fingers will run along the sides of her vaginal wall, an area seldom touched in common fingering positions, and thus, something likely to be a bit new and exciting for your lady.

Cervix

The cervix (Latin for "neck") of the uterus (cylindrical or conical in shape) is the narrow part that protrudes slightly into the vagina, leaving a circular recess around its base. Approximately half its length is available to be touched or massaged; the remainder lies above the vagina and beyond access. The front part of this recess is called the anterior fornix. Pressure on it produces rapid vaginal lubrication, even in women who are not normally sexually responsive.

The cervix will feel like a slippery cone about an inch in diameter (slightly oval, actually) and usually less than an inch in height. If you fold your index finger into the palm of your hand, the shape of your knuckle will give you a rough idea of what you should expect to find. Please note that the cervix can be found in somewhat different places among different women. Also, her enjoyment of cervix play may change depending upon where she is in her menstrual cycle.

> **Tip #9:** With your lady on her back, if you insert your third and fourth fingers, you can probably get under her cervix. This is a very sensitive spot, and this action pleases most women. While there, catch the cervix between those two fingers and massage it, starting at the point where it connects to the vaginal wall and then squeezing gently until your fingers slide off the end. NOTE: Women who have had hysterectomies no longer have a cervix.

Erogenous Hot Spots

In addition to the vaginal passage and its surrounding labia, the female genitals also boast four sexual hot spots. These are small zones where a woman feels somewhat greater sensitivity than is found in the surrounding areas. Generally, people find that stimulating these areas during sexual play can help to bring the lady to orgasm.

These areas are:

Outside the vagina

- Clitoris
- U-spot

Inside the vagina

- G-spot, and
- A-spot

(I know, I'd never heard of the U-spot or the A-spot, either. I came upon them as I began researching this book. But they're fun to play with. Ditto for differentiating between the "G" and the "A" spots. Even if the lady can't tell you which one you're on, the exploration is a lot of good fun.)

Outside the Vagina

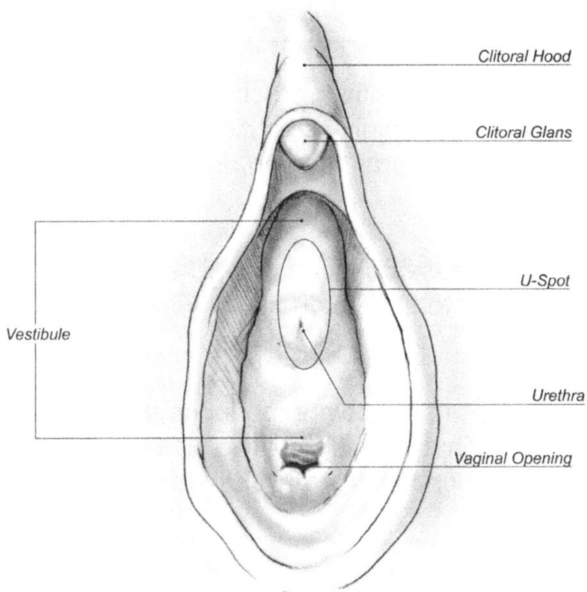

Clitoris: The clitoris comes in a wide array of sizes — from very small to quite prominent. Generally, the clitoris is thought only to be a small white oval at the end of the clitoral shaft. That's not quite right. What is commonly called the clitoris (clit, for short) is, in fact, a small body of spongy tissue that is really the clitoral glans; the reason it is highly sexually sensitive is that it contains something like 30,000 nerve endings.

In fact, there is quite a bit more to the clitoral network than merely the glans. If you want to learn about female genital anatomy in great detail, I strongly endorse The Clitoral Truth by Rebecca Chalker. This book really helped me to understand the specific parts of a woman.

Anyway, the clitoral shaft is protected by the clitoral hood, which is attached to the glans, just underneath the surface of the skin. The shaft is a round fibrous segment of spongy erectile tissue that extends 4-6 inches into her body, and like the glans, is very sensitive.

> **Tip #10:** If you roll your finger back and forth just above the glans during sexual play, you should be able to feel a hard ridge about one-half to one inch long (it extends many inches into the woman's body). While its diameter varies among women, that's the clitoral shaft. Many ladies love it when you roll your index finger back and forth over it. Similarly, you can catch the shaft between your thumb and finger and stoke down on it (towards the clit) and win her real appreciation.

U-spot: The urethral spot (U-spot) is a small patch of sensitive (erectile) tissue found just *above* and on either side of the urethral opening. This is a highly specific area of sensitivity; most (but not all) ladies are less sensitive *below* the urethral opening down to the vaginal opening.

This is a fairly recent discovery by American clinical research workers. They found that if this region was gently caressed (with your finger, your tongue, or the tip of your penis) there often was a pleasant erotic response.

Not intending to throw ice water on this discovery, it is my own experience that this area of sensitivity is exactly reversed for some women. That is, the sensitive skin is below, not above, the urethral opening. But, that's why it's so much fun to learn what does and doesn't work for a specific lady.

By the way, in books about sex, the overall area above the vaginal opening and ending just below the clitoral glans is often described and called the *vestibule.* As that area includes the patch of skin now termed the "U-spot," it is my suspicion is that this is an area well-known for its erotic potential, but only recently isolated and described by the medical community.

Inside the Vagina

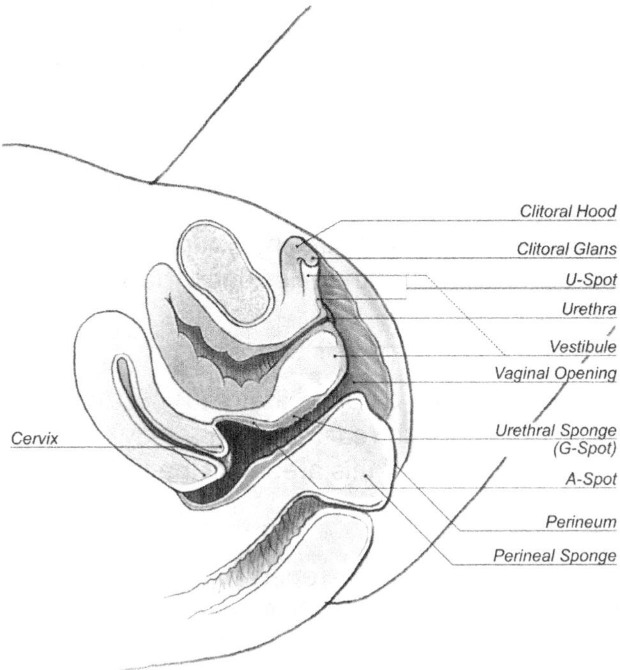

G-spot: First identified in 1981, the hotly-debated Gräfenberg spot, or G-spot, is said to be an area located within the spongy tissue that is found on the front wall of the vagina, very slightly below the surface and about two inches in from the vaginal opening (see illustration). Size varies among women. According to Gräfenberg, spongy tissue starts to swell (and pulse) with arousal. The size of the G-spot is unrelated to its sensitivity. He says that this area becomes a primary erogenous zone that may be more important than the clitoris. As there is so much conflicting information about the G-spot, I'll simply suggest you do your own research. By the way, you might want to try an Internet search on topics such as *G-spot and sexual positions.* There appear to be a very limited number of positions in which your penis can stimulate her G-spot.

> **Tip #11:** Generally, you can't touch this area with your penis when you're in the missionary position because of the physical location of the spongy tissue. That's one of the key reasons why the material in this book can be so pleasing to a lady; unless you're used to playing with her G-spot, the kind of play described here may give her some nice, new sensations.
>
> On the other hand, if you are/were used to controlling your angle of your penis' entry, you *can* hit the A-spot from the missionary position, so she may not be missing much.

On a practical level, the authors of many sex books propose that you must press deeply into the spongy tissue with two fingers to obtain much reaction from a lady. Personally, I stay well away from any deep or vigorous massaging of this area until the lady is extremely aroused.

Research seems to indicate that about half of all women report the G-spot to be highly sensitive and, under the right conditions, feels very pleasurable when stimulated. For some women, it can be a primary source of stimulation leading to orgasm during fingering and/ or during some intercourse positions. Other women report no particular sensation. In my experience, women who have not had much experience with female ejaculation start out by saying that pressing on the spongy tissue makes them feel as though they need to urinate (for which reason you might encourage your playmate to urinate before playing). As you can see from any representation of internal female organs, when you're pulling up on the G-spot, you're also putting pressure on her bladder — so her sensation is quite real.

As I just mentioned, the G-spot is often linked to the phenomenon known as female ejaculation. To date, there is little data about female ejaculation, although there appears to be growing consensus that it is the product of the Skene's glands. You'll find greater detail on this subject in Chapter Four.

A-spot

This area is a relatively new discovery, if "discovery" is the right term. This spot seems to have first been reported by a Malaysian physician in the 1990s; he also referred to it as the Epicenter. In Western medicine, it seems to be referred to as the AFE-zone (Anterior Fornix Erogenous Zone).

This A-spot is a patch of sensitive tissue in the vaginal canal between the cervix and the urethral sponge. It is described technically as the female degenerated prostate. In other words, it is the female equivalent of the male prostate, just as the clitoris is the female equivalent of the male penis. Direct stimulation at the correct time of female arousal, can produce violent orgasmic contractions. Unlike the clitoris, it is not supposed to suffer from post-orgasmic over-sensitivity. At this writing, it can be hard to find a vibrator that is designed to hit this area. You should be looking for a toy that is long and thin, with a tip that has a short 90-degree bend in it. Most currently on the market have a short 45-degree bend.

Concluding Note

According to Desmond Morris (a world-renowned British zoologist, author, and painter), "Students of female sexual physiology claim (perhaps over-enthusiastically) that if these four erotic centers are stimulated in rotation, one after the other, it is possible for a woman to enjoy many orgasms in a single night. It is pointed out, however, that it takes an extremely experienced and sensitive lover to achieve this." (Morris, Desmond. The Naked Woman: A Study of the Female Body. London: Jonathan Cape, 2004)

Chapter Summary

This chapter was devoted to identifying the sexual parts of a woman. I began by reviewing female genitalia, and then progressed to a discussion of female sexual hot spots. This discussion included the erogenous hot spots divided into those that are inside and those that are outside the vagina: the clitoris, the U-spot, the G-spot, and the A-spot.

Chapter Four

Concerning Stimulation and Ejaculation

Notes on Female Ejaculation

According to Wikipedia, "Female ejaculation, known colloquially as squirting or gushing, refers to the expulsion of noticeable amounts of clear fluid by human females from the urethra during orgasm." (Wikipedia's entries change over time, as it can be altered by any reader. This is the way it appeared on July 2, 2007.)

Before I take on a discussion of the details of female ejaculation, I'd like to register my objection to the Wikipedia definition. In my personal experience, female ejaculation and female orgasm are separate issues and occur at different times during an evening of sexual play. I'll go into more detail in a couple of pages.

Back, now to discussing female ejaculation.

Recent research (2002) suggests that the Skene's glands are the source of female ejaculation. The Skene's glands are in the general area of the urethral opening and are similar to the male prostate. They drain into the urethra near the urethral opening. In fact, the milky fluid that emerges during female ejaculation is sometimes compared in composition to the fluid generated in males by the prostate gland. (In men, the prostate gland produces the watery component of semen.)

But this news comes with a somewhat shocking footnote from the Italian researcher Emanuele Jannini of L'Aquila University, Italy, who initially propounded this theory. He has proposed that this liquid was coming from the Skene's gland openings, as opposed to the urethral opening, although more recent research suggests that the Skene's glands may also drain into the urethra. These little openings are usually the size of pinholes, but vary in size from one woman to another, to the point that they appear to be missing entirely in some women. In these instances, female ejaculation becomes anatomically impossible.

Jannini goes on to point out that if Skene's glands are, indeed, the cause of female ejaculation — and that some women have very small, or no, Skene's glands — this can explain why some women can't ejaculate. He also mentions that retrograde ejaculation, where the fluid travels up the urethra towards the bladder, could also possibly account for the absence of visible ejaculate in some women.

Ongoing Confusion

Jannini's research aside, some studies seem to point toward female ejaculate as being expelled through the urethra. However, this confusion could result from the fact that the Skene's glands are located on either side of the urethral opening — so it's easy to understand how this confusion could have occurred prior to the discovery of the function of the Skene's glands. Other current (non-medical) writers on this topic continue to believe that the fluid leaves the body through the vagina. Personally, I've seen many, many clips on the Internet showing copious amounts of fluid apparently being emitted from the woman's vagina. However, these are not close-up clips, and they certainly are not intended to settle any clinical research questions. That said, in my own experience, when my hand is in a woman's vagina and she ejaculates, I certainly feel the fluid hitting the palm of my hand that's folded over her entire vulva. That means that the fluid is coming from a source above her vagina. If the fluid were coming out her vagina, it would have to flow over the backs of my fingers, and that's not what's happening.

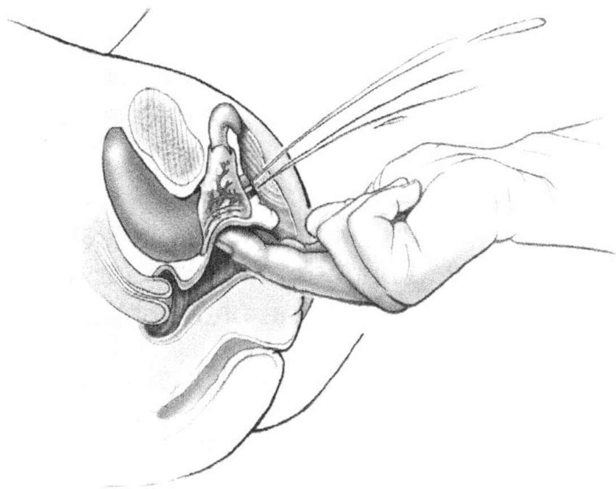

Some skeptical medical responses to the question of female ejaculation try to explain it away by considering the woman to have an infection. At that point, they call the discharge *profuse vaginal discharge.* They then say that this symptom can have different causes. They start out by stating that the infection (whether or not sexually transmitted) is usually accompanied by symptoms including itching, odor, and/or redness. Additionally, they say, a sexually transmitted infection such as *Trichomonas vaginalis* will often be present without typical symptoms of an infection, yet may be identified through a much greater than normal discharge with no other symptoms. (As these examples seem to be reporting discharge relating from various kinds of infections, I don't understand how they get cited in a paper discussing female ejaculation unless the physicians are so convinced that there is no such thing as female ejaculation that they simply switch the subject to infection-induced vaginal discharge.)

Continuing with the medical warning, it is for this reason that it is important that any female who experiences abnormal amounts of vaginal discharge undergo a physical examination to rule out underlying medical conditions. In other cases, warn the researchers, women who may not be properly educated about female ejaculation may assume that they are experiencing urinary stress incontinence and will go to their doctor. Treatment for urinary stress incontinence will often involve the use of medications or surgery that are both unnecessary and dangerous if the source of the fluid is actually female ejaculate. Before going to the doctor, a lady should try to determine whether the fluid is female ejaculate (generally colorless and odorless), urine, or something else. Ejaculation would happen only during the course of sexual play, so should be easy to distinguish from other discharges. Anyway, stress incontinence (urination) can happen during coughing, sneezing, or heavy lifting — just to add another dimension to this discussion.

More Detail for Readers Who Are Hopelessly Compulsive

Women who expel fluid during orgasm report the color, smell, consistency, and even taste, vary from one occurrence to the next, sometimes even within one sexual episode. Research also indicates that while it is safe for a woman to taste her own ejaculate, and that is also safe for the male member of a fluid bonded pair to taste the liquid, it is **not safe** for couples who are practicing safer sex (that is, not fluid bonded, thus wearing a condom during intercourse). The reason it's only safe for a fluid bonded man to taste the ejaculate of his fluid bonded partner is that female ejaculate is a body fluid, thus a potential carrier of sexually transmitted infections. (Of course, being fluid bonded has nothing to do with whether or not either party already has STIs; once fluid bonded, the presumption is that you've already been as exposed as you're going to be.)

There are reports from some women that their menstrual cycle influences the smell/taste/consistency of expelled fluid. Also, the nature of the ejaculate can be influenced both by the lady's diet and by how much liquid she consumed before you started your evening. Some women report it is sometimes clear and odorless and other times, thick and pungent.

> **Tip #12:** Female ejaculate should be fairly colorless and almost odorless. If you get urine, that will be perfectly obvious both from the smell and the color. Expelling urine rather than ejaculate is attributed to women who are trying too hard to ejaculate (to please the man?).

Creams for Increasing Female Arousal

A number of creams have been developed to aid female arousal. In my experience, those available in drug stores tend to smell medicinal, and you probably won't feel like getting any in your mouth. On the other hand, once you start looking at creams available online (try a search for *creams for female arousal*) or in sex stores, you'll find many choices. As it's inappropriate to specify my own preference, I will simply say that it comes in about six flavors and costs less than $10 per jar.

By the way, some creams contain the amino acid Arginine, purported to increase blood flow (this amino acid is also found in many male erection products). Arginine is claimed to increase sensations and enhance orgasms.

> **Safety Warning #1:** Be cautious about any stimulant that purports to increase a woman's estrogen level. Estrogen is known to feed certain types of cancer, such as breast cancer. High estrogen levels in women can increase cancerous growth.

G-spot Play

What Is the G-spot? Where Is the G-spot?

The female prostate and the Gräfenberg spot (G-spot) are **not** the same thing, nor are they located in the same place. Recall our discussion about the A-spot, above. The G-spot is a non-specific area of tissue on the lady's spongy tissue that becomes accessible once the spongy tissue becomes engorged with blood during arousal.

The problem with any definition of the G-spot is that research physicians can find no anatomical structure that can clearly be named the G-spot. This may explain why so many men (and women) have trouble finding it and why there is so much urban legend surrounding it.

At any rate, the G-spot's sensitivity — and even its existence — differs from woman to woman. Here's what I've found from researching the topic:

- If a woman is not sexually aroused, she may not have a locatable G-spot.
- If the same woman is highly aroused, and her spongy tissue is engorged, she may have a very distinct G-spot — but not necessarily in exactly the same place you found it before.
- Some women are not aware of a G-spot, even though they may have intense orgasms, and even though they may ejaculate when this area is sufficiently stimulated.

Because of this wide variation between women, readers should not form a fixed idea of what a G-spot is or where it is located. Each woman creates her own definition that is valid only for her.

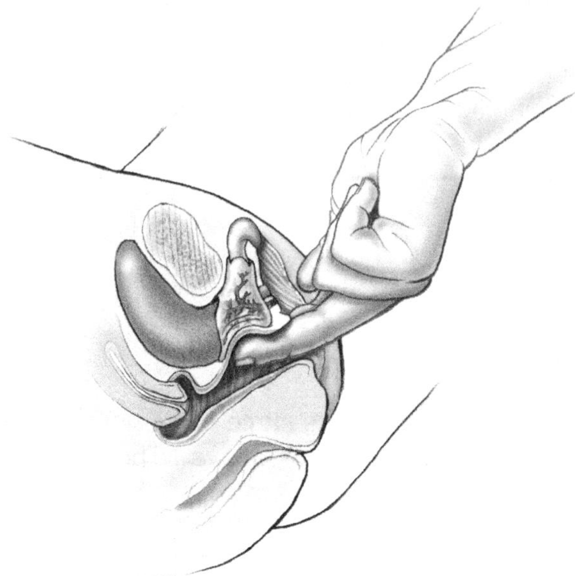

The greatest known female ejaculate-evokers are the A-spot and the G-spot. Stroking and rubbing either place, using techniques I'll cover in this book, should get you there — so long as the woman actually *has* Skene's glands that come through to the surface of her skin (discussed earlier).

Many women who have experienced orgasms both from clitoral stimulation and from G-spot manipulation claim that it is easier to have multiple G-spot orgasms than it is to have multiple clitoral orgasms. If you are able to induce an episode of ejaculation with your lady — not necessarily associated with an orgasm, by the way — continue what you were doing that produced the female ejaculation. You may well be rewarded with multiple ejaculations. Depending upon the woman, and depending upon how hydrated she is, three, four or even five episodes are not uncommon.

Orgasms and Ejaculation

In Women

These events are generally well separated in time. In my experience, women ejaculate separately from their orgasms; with practice, you can easily manage/control this difference through sequencing your own techniques. Also, you may well find women who climax and ejaculate simultaneously.

In Men

As in women, orgasms and ejaculations can be separate events for men. However, this appears not to be well-known in Western cultures. There are courses of study (and books written) about the exercises needed to separate the two. The two books that come most to mind are these:

- Keesling, Barbara. How to Make Love All Night (and Drive a Woman Wild). New York: Harper Collins, 1994, and

- McNeil, James W. Ancient Lovemaking Secrets: The Journey Toward Immortality. L9H Publishers, 1998.

With that as prologue, at some point in your life, your body may stop producing testosterone. Although testosterone loss varies among men, in a general sense, young men can sustain many ejaculations in one evening and older men cannot. In some men (myself included), testosterone loss is dramatically noticeable; rather like turning off a switch. One day you'll have no problems with ejaculate recovery, the next day practically nothing will be going on. A trip to your primary care physician (after a blood work-up) should give you medical confirmation about your testosterone level. When you lose your testosterone, a number of things may happen:

- You may lose sexual interest in women.

- You may have a harder time getting an erection and maintaining it.

- You may not be able to ejaculate as often, and once you do, it may take *much* longer to build up to another ejaculation.

You may conclude that you'll need to start taking a testosterone hormone replacement in addition to prescription or non-prescription erectile dysfunction pills.

> **Tip #13:** Prescription and non-prescription erection enhancers affect only a man's ability to have and maintain an erection. They have nothing to do with a man's ability to ejaculate. These are separate issues that must be treated separately.

The level of testosterone in the man's body has everything to do with his ability to ejaculate (and the speed with which the man's body can recover to ejaculate a second or third time) and much less to do with erections. It also has a great deal to do with your interest in having sex. Low testosterone levels = low interest in sex. It's like you just stop thinking about it.

This is because testosterone is the hormone that affects your libido; your libido affects lots of other things about you. If you're interested in doing further research on this topic, Wikipedia may be a good place to start.

So, men, as you age and find you are having problems either with the hardness of your erection or with the frequency of your ejaculations, please understand that they are separate issues that need to be discussed with your physician. As there is no cure for this condition, you must consult your physician about management strategies. Due to drug pricing, among other things, you might wish to consider a combination of prescription and non-prescription medications — but only with your physician's knowledge and approval.

Before leaving this section, I want to bring up another cause for erection difficulties. In many cases, erection issues are psychological, rather than physiological. That is, something other than simply having a naked woman in front of you is required for you to get an erection. As I discuss in the section on *cleanliness and fetishes* (Chapter Ten), sometimes men get sexually aroused by different things. That said, some common fetishes could be found in a man's response to:

- Breasts
- Vulva
- Rear end
- Certain types of dress/clothing (think garter belt and hose or dressy latex)
- Bondage
- Giving measured pain
- Receiving measured pain

In fact, there are hundreds and hundreds of sexual fetishes. If you care to spend some time looking at them, see: http://public.diversity.org.uk/deviant/dictindx.htm. Internet searches will also bring up interesting (and often anxiety-reducing) results.

Chapter Summary

This chapter opened with a discussion of female ejaculation and some of the confusion that surrounds it. I then provided a quick review of other causes of vaginal discharge, indicating that female ejaculate was distinctive because of its relative odorlessness. I mentioned that you might try a cream for increasing female arousal, and then discussed the G-spot and the role it plays with orgasm and ejaculation. I ended with a discussion about how erections and ejaculation in men (and women) are separable events.

Part III

Toys

Chapter Five

Lubes

Caution: Avoid lubes with the ingredient nonoxynol-9. It is very irritating to many women. (Source: Ultimate Guide to Cunnilingus, p 57). Here is an additional comment on spermicides and condoms from the Toys in Babeland website (www.toysinbabeland.com):

"Nonoxynol-9 is effective as a spermicide, but many people don't know that it is a detergent that can irritate sensitive tissues and actually promote the spread of STIs. Condoms lubricated with nonoxynol-9 have not been proven more effective in preventing pregnancy than regular lubricated condoms. If you, or a partner, are irritated by nonoxynol-9, consider using regular condoms with extra lube from a bottle."

The Major Categories of Lubes

Lubes come in these general categories:

- Water-based
- Vegetable-based
- Oil-based
- Silicone-based
- Specialty Lubes
- Alternatives to Lubes

The type of lube that you use depends on whether you're heading for her vagina or her anus. It also depends upon whether you intend to use the lube in conjunction with a latex condom or a silicone toy. It also depends upon whether she's prone to yeast infections.

> **Safety Warning #2:** Lubes and the vagina: Remember, you're dealing with an area that stays warm and wet 100% of the time. Enclosed + warm + wet = microbial growth chamber. Think yeast infection. Think unhappy playmate. It's a good general rule to avoid putting anything sweet in there. No lollypops, no ice cream, no whipped cream, no glycerin-based lubes. Water-based, only. Be sure to check the label to verify that the manufacturer didn't slip a little glycerin into lube that's supposed to be water-based.

Water-based

Water-based personal lubricants are water-soluble and are generally less irritating to body surfaces than any alternative lube. These water-based lubes are relatives of a cellulose and water combination, originally labeled Surgilube® and released in the 1950s. According to my research, subsequent products have added a variety of agents for spreading, for water retention, or to increase resistance to contamination. They have a tendency to dry out during use, but can be reactivated by adding water; they also can be thinned by adding water.

Since the 1980s, a few companies have produced a water-soluble, silicon co-polymer (dimethicone) for a prolonged slippery effect. While these contain a silicone component, they are still water-based products. They are very slippery. While this is great if you're playing with sex toys, this can be a disadvantage when it comes to intercourse, because a certain amount of friction is necessary for optimal sensation. If your water-based lube contains silicone, its viscosity cannot be adjusted. Also, they can stain both clothing and sheets.

If you're planning on having intercourse in water, water-based lubricants won't work; that kind of lube will simply dissolve or disperse in water.

Popular brands include K-Y Jelly®, Wet®, and Astroglide®.

Vegetable-based

Vegetable-based lubes are primarily used for anal, not vaginal fisting. According to those who know such things, Crisco™ used to be the main choice for that activity because it's cheap, easily obtainable, and ready in an instant. Also, because it's so cheap, you can discard a can after one use — a health issue. The problems are that it's messy, hard to clean up, and has a peculiar "Mom's baking in the kitchen" smell that many object to.

Oil-based

According to Answers.com (http://www.answers.com/topic/personal-lubricant): "Unlike water-based lubricants, oil-based lubricants, such as Vaseline®, dissolve latex and are likely to reduce the effectiveness of latex condoms as a contraceptive and protection against sexually transmitted infections. Oil-based lubricants should never be used either for anal sex or vaginal sex, as the oil may coat the lining of the opening, providing a haven for bacterial infection."

Although petroleum jelly (i.e. Vaseline®), baby oil, and mineral oil are all inexpensive and readily available, they're not water-soluble. As you should not introduce soaps or shampoos into the vaginal canal, it would be very hard to clean the woman after using products such as these as lubes.

Silicone-based

Technically, most silicone-based lubricants are oils; water won't break them down. They tend to retain lubrication longer than water-based lubricants.

Silicone-based lubricants probably should not be used with silicone-based sex toys. I'll discuss this again, but there appears to be some degradation of silicone sex toys by silicone lubes. However, silicone lubes work very well with latex condoms. As an aside, you may actually find that you prefer a plastic condom such as Durex's Avanti®. Many men feel that plastic condoms such as these transfer heat and sensation better than latex condoms, so there's an added incentive. They are also a good alternative for those with latex allergies.

Anyway, popular brands of silicone-based lubes include Eros Bodyglide®, Wet Platinum Premium Body Glide®, DeGLOW®, and System Jo® (System Jo comes in a number of versions — 100% silicone and also in a water-soluble version — which is my personal choice).

Specialty Lubes

Specialty lubricants are designed to cause localized changes, including increased blood flow (creating a fuller erection of the penis or clitoris) or warming. Other lubes include flavors along with slipperiness. Popular brands include Wet® fun flavors (warming), KY Jelly® (warming) and Thermal® (warming vasodilator).

Safety Warning #3: Before purchasing a lube containing vasodilating and or sensitivity maximizing ingredients, please remember always to check the label for ingredients to which you might have allergies or sensitivities. Also, if you are on prescription medications, check with your doctor or pharmacist for possible drug interactions. If you experience any itching, burning, redness, or rash, stop using the product immediately and check with your doctor. Follow the directions on the package.

Alternatives to Lubes

A Wikipedia search on "personal lubricants" produced this interesting chart. Although I considered simply sending you to the website, I decided that it should be included here, as it's interesting and includes alternatives I'd never thought about. Again, this is taken from Wikipedia (a free-use website) and is not the product of my personal research.

Safety Warning #4: The use of food as a lubricant is contra-indicated for hygienic reasons. All foods carry either a common mostly harmless pathogen and/or contribute to the cultivation of pathogens.

Improvised Lubricant	***Type***	***Notes***
Saliva	Water-based	This is 98% water and may contain irritating levels of acidic electrolytes and gastric juices.
Vegetable gums		This is more than 95% water, plus vegetable gum (e.g.: Xantham gum). It is edible. Most commercial lubricants contain some type of gum.
Egg white		About 83% water, 10% protein and less than 7% fat (Pathogen content depends on the food handling safety of the farms, the transportation systems, and the supermarkets).
Banana filling	Oil and/ or Water-based	These vary in percentage of water and may contain dehydrating levels of sugars/salts, and irritating levels of allergens, acids (citric acid, ascorbic acid) etc. (Pathogen content depends on the food handling safety of the farms, the transportation systems, the supermarkets, and individual kitchens).
Baba ghanoush		
Pie filling		
Tahini		
Butter (fairly slippery, but oily. Not usually toxic if fresh. Will support some micro-organisms.)		
Caviar (only for the rich)		Only James Bond would do this, and I'm confident that he would want the lady stirred, not shaken. No, this wasn't in the original Wikipedia chart, but we couldn't miss the opportunity to add it.
Moisturizing body lotion	Oil-based	Any medication content can cause harmful side effects and cause antibiotic-resistant bacterial strains to evolve. It is even possible that they can become lethal.
Mineral oil		If used orally, it should be swallowed with care, as it works as a laxative within six hours. If aspirated into the lungs, it can cause lipoid pneumonia.
Cooking oil		As above, and it also can increase your risk of bacterial infection (e.g.: dipping fingers into the container will cause contamination and cultivation).

Relevant note: Perhaps the best-known, non-specialized lubricant is a make-up cleanser called Albolene.

Matching the Lube With Your Play

It's easy to get confused about the interactions between lubes and safer sex supplies and/or sex toys. To simplify, there are two interactions to remember:

Latex and Oil-based Products

Oils and fats (called *lipids*) will degrade latex. "Degrade" is the euphemism for "melt." You would be surprised how fast that can happen. For a demonstration, take a latex condom or latex glove and stick it in some Crisco™ and set it aside for a while. Although the time it takes to dissolve will vary with the manufacturer of the glove or condom, the results should be about the same: deterioration over time.

"Okay," you say, "I promise not to rub Crisco™ all over my partner and contaminate my condom." Fine, but what about massage oils? Same problem, slower effect. Slow enough that you don't have to worry about it? I have no idea; it depends upon the latex manufacturer and the type of oil you're using.

So, if you're massaging your partner with oil and reach for latex or jelly dildos or butt-toys, you risk degrading the latex. In the case of condoms, that can lead to their failure. If you want more detailed information about which toys can and cannot be used with oil-based lubes, check them out on www.goodvibes.com. They have extensive material on this topic.

Silicone Lubes and Silicone Toys

It appears that silicone lubes are 100% latex safe, so you don't have to worry about condoms breaking (at least, not from that). However, while silicone lubes can be safely used with **some** silicone toys, it appears that they can't be used with *all* silicone toys.

Confusing, yes? Here's what Good Vibrations (www.goodvibes.com) has to say about silicone interaction:

"...the makers of some silicone sex toys have indicated that silicone lubes can degrade silicone sex toys with extended use. Reports on this interaction are mixed, and it may be that silicone lubes are safe with some silicone sex toys and not with others. But to be on the safe side, we suggest that you avoid using this combination. And if you use condoms on your silicone dildos and butt-toys (a great idea, by the way, both for easy cleanup and safer sex), do be aware that many lubricated condoms use some sort of silicone-based lube. So we definitely advise you to use non-lubricated condoms for this purpose.

"If you wish to be ultra-safe, we recommend using a water-based lube; water-based lubes have no bad interactions with either latex or silicone."

A Few Ending Notes

A drop of lube on the head of a penis before applying a condom will make the tip of the condom slip back and forth over the penis head, thus increasing the man's sensitivity during intercourse. But beware; putting too much lube *inside* the condom will cause the condom to come off during intercourse.

In the "for what it's worth" department, the frothy mixture of lube and fecal matter that is sometimes the byproduct of anal sex is called santorum.

> **Safety Warning #5:** Be particularly cautious where this santorum goes. As previously noted, you don't want to get any fecal matter in the vaginal area. Bad safety risk.

Chapter Summary

This chapter has reviewed the major categories of lubes: water-based, vegetable-based, oil-based, silicon-based, specialty lubes, and alternatives to lubes. I provided pros and cons of each type of lube, including suggestions about which lube to use for the kind of play you're intending. The most basic warning is that you want to avoid using lubes containing sugar (glucose, sucrose, fructose) in the vagina. I pointed out that *oil-based lubes* are likely to degrade latex gloves, condoms, and latex toys, and that while *silicone lubes* are latex-safe, they seem to degrade some, but not all, silicone toys.

Chapter Six

Vibrators and Such

Safety Warning #6: If you're playing sexually with multiple partners with whom you are not fluid bonded, and if you're playing with vibrators that have a porous surface (such as plastic, rubber, or silicone toys), you ***must*** cover them with a condom. You must do this to avoid the possibility of contaminating them with body fluids that could contain STIs. Many sex toys can retain body fluids unless you're disinfecting them with some kind of medical cleanser (see *Cleaning your Sex Toys,* below).

Opening Notes

Some Negative Personal Views About Vibrators and Dildos

Some women hold strong views about using vibrators — and even dildos — that men need to be aware of. There are those of both genders who love them, and there are those of both genders who avoid them. As this chapter is about ways of pleasing a lady with vibrators, I'd like to present some comments from ladies who *don't* like them. These bullets are a summary of responses I received after polling about 30 women. I've restructured their answers to fit the writing style of this book.

- "I don't want a man using a vibrator on me. That's too private, too personal. I use a vibrator to masturbate in my own bedroom. I'd be embarrassed if a man used one on me."
- "If I've got a man around, I want the *man*, not some substitute."
- "I have a very dominant personality. I love vibrators, but I'll only allow another dominant man to use them on me. If the man is of a submissive sort, it would feel completely wrong."
- "Vibrators are *plastic!* They are hard, often cold, and usually covered in face slime (aka lube). For as much as they are intended to hit the G-spot in such a good way, put one in the wrong hands and it hits the most tender spots with an unforgiving force that downright hurts! Nothing will get me OUT of the mood faster. And yeah, try explaining to the person at the controls that they "took a wrong turn in there." I have yet to find a respectful, appreciative, adoring way of saying, 'Yeow! That hurts. Get that thing out of me RIGHT NOW.'"
- "Well, I do like vibrators, but not so much the dildo-only vibrators. I'm very much the clit stimulation girl. As much as I love the feel of being filled, beyond that I don't get much out of vaginal vibrators. If a dildo/vibrator is inserted and kept there for a long period of time it actually starts to hurt."
- "No, I don't like vibrators used on me. This isn't because I don't like vibrators — they are awesome tools — but I feel there are many women who become addicted to them, because it's so much easier to get to climax, so much easier to get the sex act over. I feel as though vibrators desensitize me, therefore making a climax/orgasm more difficult to achieve naturally. (By that I mean using my muscles and breathing to achieve climax.) Not using vibrators is a choice for me."
- "I was non-orgasmic with partners, and the thought of having a vibrator reveal, on the one hand, how disappointedly and humiliatingly non-orgasmic I was in front of another, or on the other hand, how unladylike and, possibly abnormal, my orgasms were, was embarrassing. So, I avoided them until quite recently. In general, I'd guess, speaking from my own experience, that a woman's discomfort with vibrators, oral sex, etc., is often based on an expectation of self-humiliation."

From the man's point of view, the most common comments I hear are some variations on the themes that they don't view *using vibrators* as a manly activity; also, they don't *need* to use vibrators when they have a penis.

I certainly understand the reluctance of some women to allow men to play with vibrators when their previous experiences have been so negative. I also understand how some ladies who are not very vaginally sensitive aren't interested in vibrating dildos. That said, I would encourage men to approach their ladies with sensitivity and understanding and demonstrate to them that you can be trusted to use vibrators in ways that will relax and please them.

In Defense of Vibrators

You can create dozens of relaxing and sexually stimulating sensations with vibrators that you can't create with any other toy — or with your penis. But they're not idiot-proof. You have to learn to use vibrators as you have to learn how to use any other tool. I've taught vibrator play for some time, and often hear a man say, "Oh, she doesn't like that one; I've tried it." Well, my guess is that he tried it without knowing how to read her reactions and modify his touch, based on those reactions. My experiences with vibrators have led me to develop some rules:

1. Don't dismiss vibrators as sex toys until you've seen what they can do.
2. Start out with very, very light touches: Tease her — and stay away from her clit at the outset. Hold off on that activity as long as you can. Build her up for clitoral play.
3. Lower vibrator speeds send sensations further into the body — don't always go for the highest speed settings on your vibrator. *Faster* vibration is seldom *better* in this case. (Think how it feels when your stereo system is playing loudly and you turn the treble down and the bass way up. Now reverse the controls and notice how you can no longer feel the musical vibrations through your body. This is why nightclubs with dance floors have the bass and the volume set so high; it is sexually arousing.)
4. For clitoral-only play, the higher the vibrating speed, the better. When you start your clitoral play, begin by grazing the clit, then go away. Then stay a little longer, then go away… You get the idea.
5. Always, always, always sanitize your toys after using them in sexual play.

A zillion makes and models of vibrators exist. There are a couple of reasons for this wide variety. First, because women respond differently, there's a vibrator out there for every preference — and more coming on the market all the time. Second, these things vibrate at different frequencies, so they evoke different responses from your lady/ladies. If you're just starting out to explore the world of vibrators, you may well end up owning a group that you use on a regular basis and another group that you can draw from once you've developed the sensitivity to play off your lady's reactions.

Vibrators are classified in two ways — those generally intended to be used **outside** her body and those generally intended to be used **inside** her body. I say generally, because there is a lot of overlap, here. Some large-head outside vibrators (such as Hitachi's Magic Wand®) can be safely inserted inside any lady that you can fist, while virtually all inside vibrators feel great when placed against your lady's outer lips, vaginal opening, and clit.

Outside Vibrators

Soft, Gentle, and Non-threatening

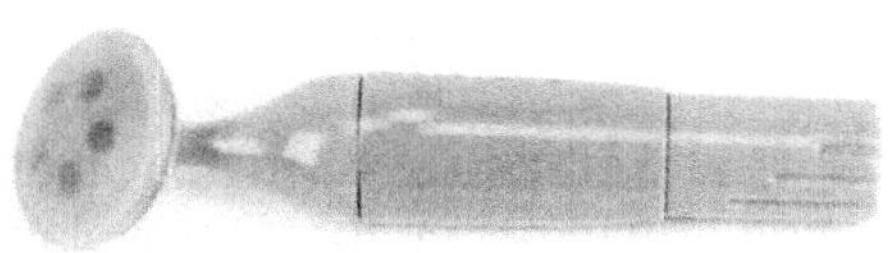

If you want to start off with a little gem that is extremely mild, I recommend one that looks like this. They're widely available and are very colorful. One model (although not the model pictured), is manufactured by Doc Johnson and is called "Jenna Velvet G®". These are inexpensive, pleasing sex toys.

Hitachi Magic Wand®

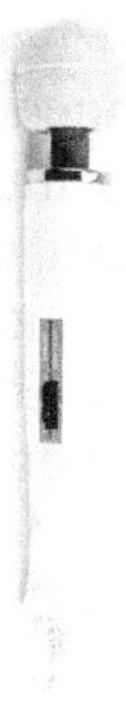

One of the most popular vibrators in the US is the Hitachi Magic Wand®. Prices vary somewhat, but you should be able to pick one up for about $50. I believe that you'll find that about 90% of the women with whom you play sexually will very quickly orgasm with this vibrator — unless you're careful. Much of the trick is slowing her down and then warming her back up.

However, there are a small percentage of women for whom the Magic Wand® is just too intense, in which case you might consider using the next item on this list.

Tip #14a: You may find that a few women who see you coming with a Magic Wand® become anxious. Some women may have had bad experiences with it. If this happens to you, ask her permission to start *very gently* by grazing her closed vulva and working up only to mild pressure before moving on to other toys. Come back to the Magic Wand® only after she's thoroughly aroused and is willing to allow you to reintroduce this vibrator. And don't get your feelings hurt if she says, "Oh, I think that's enough, thanks." Not all toys are for all women.

Tip #14b: When using this sex toy with multiple partners, you must tie a latex or non-latex condom over the vibrating head, or risk contaminating the Wand's head with body fluids. I recommend that you purchase a condom meant for men with very wide penises. (For example, one manufacturer labels these oversized condoms *Magnum.*)

In a pinch, you can also tie a non-latex glove over the head of your Hitachi. You do this by sitting down with the Wand between your knees and slipping the glove over its head. Using the glove's baby finger and thumb, tie the glove off below head. The other fingers will now be out of the way and the head of the Wand is "gloved." As soon as you try it, this will make terrific sense.

Wahl 7-in-1®

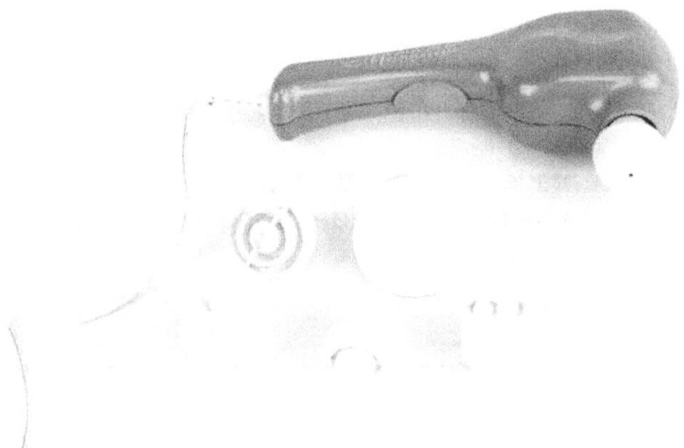

I think that as you try the Hitachi and the Wahl, you'll find that because the vibrating characteristics of these two vibrators are quite different, women seem to prefer one over the other, with not much overlap. Because of this, you'll probably need both vibrators. Women who find the Hitachi too intense are generally happier with the Wahl. Similarly, if the woman is yawning at the Wahl, try the Hitachi.

Both of these coil-operated devices have two speeds. The Wahl has both higher and a lower vibrating frequencies than the Magic Wand®. Depending on which of the seven heads you attach to it — and which of the vibrating speeds you select — the Wahl provides either a more focused or more spread-out vibrating sensation. Also, the Wahl is purported to be the quietest electric vibrator on the market. It is only 6½" long, and is easy to take on vacations or over to your date's house. (I once ran into a lady who reported that over the past decade, she had burned out three or four Wahls from extensive use, and that it was about the only vibrator she would use. I was impressed. She had two with her that evening. Don't ask. I have no idea. My only guess was that the second one was an emergency backup — rather like a professional photographer carrying two cameras. We all have our own idiosyncrasies.)

Back to the Magic Wand® for a second. Two paragraphs ago, I casually mentioned that some women find the Hitachi too intense. I've had this come up a number of times. If this applies to you, try placing a small washcloth over the entire area and try it again and lighten up on the pressure that you're using. Usually, this solves the problem.

Tongue Joy®

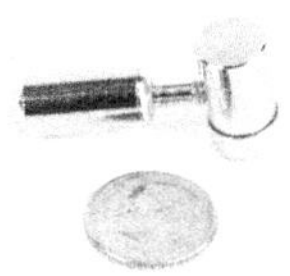

Another nice clitoral vibrator is called the Tongue Joy®. It has two principal attributes: first, it vibrates *extremely* fast (the fastest in my own collection of vibrators) and it's very, very small. I've found that this vibrator is well-received by the ladies, who often ask to have it applied again and again.

While the Tongue Joy® is extremely small, that can also be its principal downside. It can be difficult to hold between your fingers — particularly if you have a large hand. Also, you probably don't want to use it as it is intended, strapped to your tongue with a little plastic band. While it's not designed to be hand-held, it **is** possible to grasp it; your partner will thank you for your trouble. This photo shows the Tongue Joy® configured to be held between your fingers. As you can see, it's about the size of a dime.

I suggest that you start out using it to encircle the clitoris, rather than right *on* the clitoris (this thing is really intense and if you start by touching it to her clitoris, she's likely to yelp.) Because yelping brings the lady into her head, this is a mood-breaker, so don't do it. You can also use it in between the inner and outer lips. Another neat trick is to use a rubber band to attach it to your finger and actually insert it. The advantage to doing this is that this little guy gives you more control for vibrating her spongy tissue (and other internal areas) than any other vibrator that I've ever found.

The Vibro Dolphin®

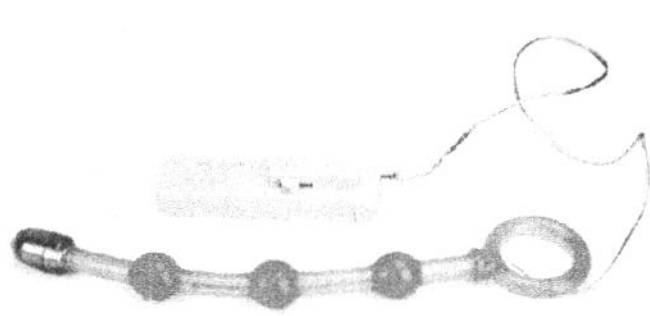

Another often-used outside vibrator is the little clit vibrator called The Vibro Dolphin®. This is a jelly-covered mini-massager with a soft jelly dolphin tickler at the top (1 AA battery); it vibrates madly. You'll want to turn the dolphin on its back and let the back touch the clit rather than the dolphin's beak. Unless, that is, you're doing adventurous sex. Anyway, it can be a lot of fun for only $10.

Inside Vibrators

Slim and Not Too Long

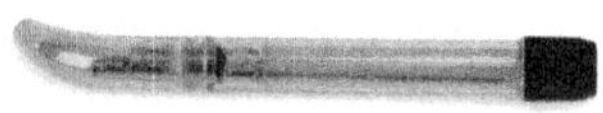

For an insertable vibrator that should be extremely non-threatening, I recommend any slim model. This one can be used either as an outside or as an inside vibrator. It has a gentle vibrating cycle — nothing too alarming. It's good for G-spot, A-spot, and for cervix stimulation. (Note: The A-spot stimulator I previously mentioned has a 90-degree bend, while this model has a 45-degree bend. However, this shape is easily purchased in this country.)

The Rimba

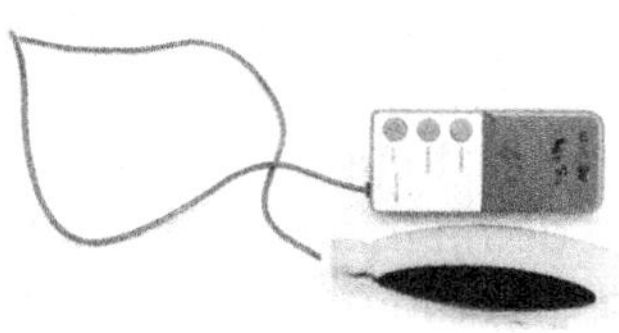

I've always found the Rimba to be popular with ladies. It has a really comfortable fit and a nice vibrating speed. Once inserted, if you grab its base, you can move it around inside your lady. It has the added advantage of (optionally) producing a very gentle electrical tickle. You'll find much more advanced sexual toys that incorporate stronger electrical stimulation (called "electrostim") if you decide to explore adventuresome sex practices.

Anal-Beads with Vibrator

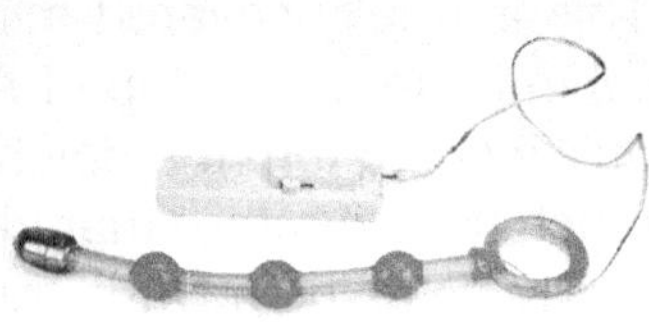

The anal-beads-with-vibrator is one of my very favorites to use on a clit because of its high vibrating frequency. It doesn't vibrate as fast as Tongue Joy®, but I think that you'll find it to be faster than most other vibrators in your collection, and — unlike the Tongue Joy® — it can be inserted either vaginally or anally (with condom). As your lady gets used to your playing with it, you may be able to push on it hard enough to make it curl back on itself — when inserted vaginally. You'll be surprised that the whole thing can fit in there. It creates a greater sense of vibration plus fullness than most vibrating dildos. You're likely to get good feedback from your ladies.

Flex-a-Pleaser®

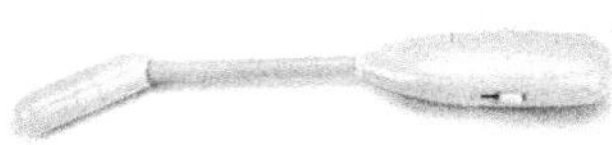

This is one of my most-used sex toys. You can start out by using it externally as a warm-up vibrator, then move on to inserting it into her vagina. If you initially inserted it so that it's pointed downward (woman on her back), rotate it upwards to vibrate over the G-spot. Hold it there. Next, rotate it 180 degrees (back to the downward position) to vibrate over the cervix. Go back and forth between these two orientations. And back and forth and back and forth and... There's plenty of room for improvisation here, so have a good time. Much later in this book, there is a discussion of how to use the Flex-a-Pleaser ® in conjunction with either the Magic Wand ® or the Wahl 7-in-1® to produce an ear-splitting orgasm.

Not Vibrators, but Interesting

Oster® Hand Massager

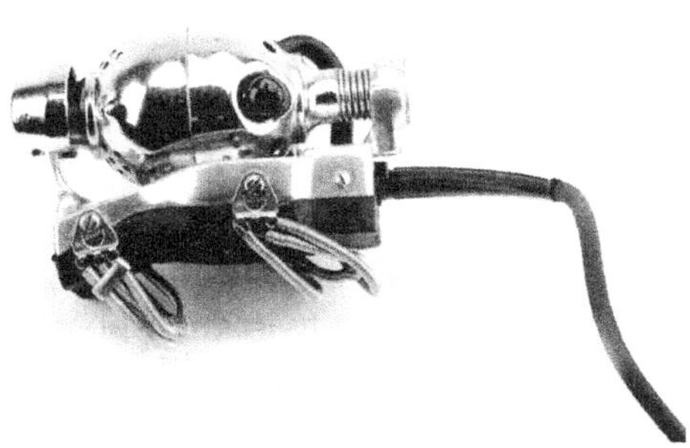

This is a "Must-Have" product. I recommend it as your first vibrator. It began life in the 1960s as a barber's vibrator. The barber would strap it to the back of his hand and massage your scalp after your haircut and before the final combing (ah, how times have changed!). It has two speed-settings, and it makes the fingers vibrate like mad. This apparatus combines high vibrating speed with the softness and warmth of your very-alive fingers.

For ladies who don't like the feel of an inorganic vibrator, this is the perfect answer. I suspect you'll use this as your starting point with most of your new sexual play partners. Oil her down, massage her back, hands, and feet with it strapped to the back of your hand. Once she's fully relaxed, ask if she would like to turn over. If she does, the world is yours.

When first introducing this vibrator, I strongly suggest that you start out using it as a scalp massager, as you'll win an instant convert to this religion. While new scalp massagers are still manufactured, there is also a brisk trade for older models on the large auction sites. The cost appears to range from $25 - $70. (As an aside, your lady can use this on you, with equally gratifying results.)

The Eroscillator®

This guy moves from side to side — thus is technically not a vibrator. So far as I know, it is the only product endorsed by Dr. Ruth. An Internet search generates lots of purchase options. They can be pricey, though, sometimes as high as $160. I've heard of people picking them up on sale in the $100 range. This vibrator comes with various interesting attachments — even a simulated mustache brush. I've spoken with some women who say this is the best vibrator they have every used; others say it's a yawn. I've never encountered a lady who sort-of liked it; it's either, "Oh gosh, *yes!*" or "Oh, gee, no thanks." The oscillating speed goes from very fast to invisibly fast.

> **Tip #15:** If your lady wishes to participate in Fabulous Sex, you might consider suggesting some pelvic floor muscle exercises and exercisers. See, for example, http://www.blowfish.com/catalog/toys/pc_exercisers.html. Women who practice tightening those muscles over a period of years can close their vaginal openings with such force that your penis is pretty well trapped. I've only known three ladies who set out to develop their PC (pubococcygeus) muscles on a daily basis. In one case, her partner (a man in his mid-30s whom I know well and trust completely) claims that if he enters her by sitting on her, she can actually capture his penis and throw him off the bed — because he can't twist out of her to balance himself. Considering he must outweigh her by 70 pounds, this is not an insignificant feat. They both think it's very funny.

Slightest Touch®

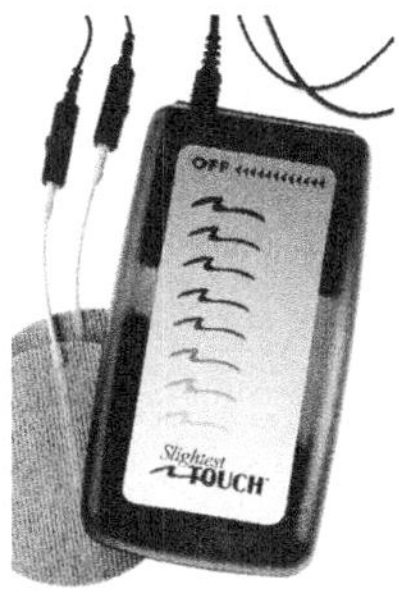

Recently, a friend of mine was telling me of a surprising new addition to his "toybag." My interest was piqued, as this particular friend is extremely sophisticated in his use of toys in sexual play, and he knows a great deal about what is called "electro-stim," the use of electricity to augment sexual play.

Over 10 years in development, Slightest Touch®, is an electrical stimulator that simulates acupuncture and is designed to do a number of very specific things to a lady:

- Magnify and intensify your existing sexual touches and techniques
- Deepen the lady's full body orgasmic response
- Hold a pre-orgasmic plateau as long as desired
- Invoke multiple and sequential orgasms

As it's not appropriate for me to personally endorse any specific product, I'll only say that it's very interesting to play with this toy, and for those of us interested in using electrical stimulation in our sex play, there's nothing else like this on the market.

Cleaning Your Sex Toys

You are responsible for maintaining a safe environment for your ladies. Because many sexually transmitted infections are carried through body fluid exchange (or through blood exchange) clean toys are a critical aspect of safe play. Here are some suggestions in that regard:

> **RelyOn™:** According to DuPont's website, this product is a tried, tested, and proven chemical disinfectant that kills 99.999% of organisms in less than 10 minutes. It is a multi-purpose disinfectant cleaner, which — when prepared as a 1% working solution — is effective against a wide range of human pathogens including Hepatitis A, B, and C, HIV, MRSA (Methicillin-resistant Staphylococcus aureus), VRE (Vanocomycin-resistant Enterococci), Influenza, and Norovirus (Norwalk-like virus).

DisCide™: DisCide™ towelettes are clinically proven to kill microorganisms on hard, inanimate, nonporous surfaces, reducing the risk of cross-contamination. It effectively kills MRSA, VRE, HIV, Herpes, Adenovirus, Staphylococcus, E-Coli, Pseudomonas, and Salmonella in one minute. It kills Trichophyton mentagrophytes in 4 minutes, and kills Staphylococcus aureus, Pseudomonas aeruginosa, and Salmonella choleraesuis in 6 minutes.

Note: RelyOn™ must be mixed; DisCide™ comes on towelettes.

Chapter Summary

I opened by recognizing that there are some negatives about vibrators, both from the male and from the female viewpoints. As some of these issues/concerns could easily affect your possible play with vibrators, I went into this subject in some detail. I asked readers to remain open to the possibility of using vibrators, as the use of vibrators is one of the most reliable techniques that I have found that can lead to screaming orgasms. I went on to review vibrators in categories: those that are used mostly outside the body, and those that are used mostly inside the body. There was a brief foray into toys not technically classified as vibrators, but that move. This chapter ended by stressing the importance of cleaning your toys; I provided two proven methods for that purpose.

Chapter Seven

Specialty Dildos

Safety Warning #6, Repeated with Slight Modification: If you're playing sexually with multiple partners with whom you are not fluid bonded, and if you're playing with dildos that have a porous surface (such as plastic, rubber, or silicone), you ***must*** cover them with a condom. You must do this to avoid the possibility of contaminating them with body fluids that could contain STIs. Many sex toys can retain body fluids unless you're disinfecting them with some kind of medical cleanser — previously discussed.

If you've already been playing with vibrating dildos for some time, then you're probably familiar with the wide range of shapes and sizes of non-vibrating dildos that are currently available. Therefore, I'm only going to touch on some of the lesser known varieties that are among my favorites.

Steel Dildos

The Probe™

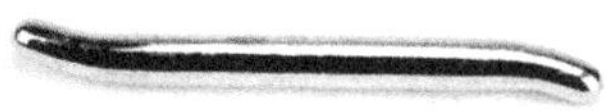

This is a pound-and-a-half of cool, sleek, solid stainless steel. At 12" long and 1.5" wide, this rod is one heck of an insertable. For the guy doing the inserting, it feels very comfortable and very heavy in your hand. You can rotate it to obtain all kinds of nice effects. By choking down on it so that only an inch or two protrudes from your fist, you can pound into her with it, simulating the feeling of your body hitting hers during intercourse. If she tells you you're hitting the back of her vaginal wall, choke it down a bit more. Hitting that back wall may also result from your lady not being sufficiently aroused. As I've mentioned, the vagina lengthens as arousal increases, often doubling its length.

If you keep The Probe™ at room temperature — say 75 degrees, and insert it into your lady's 98-degree body, she'll scream. Which may well be the point, right? (Ahem, er... moving right along...) Really, you should warm it in warm tap water. In this case, you'll want to put a thermometer in the water you're using to warm the Probe™, so you'll know when you reach body temperature. Failure to follow these directions may earn you a scream that is likely to sound a lot like STOP THAT! Anyway, the Probe™ costs about $40 from Rainbow Rope.

The Fun Wand® and the Pure Wand®

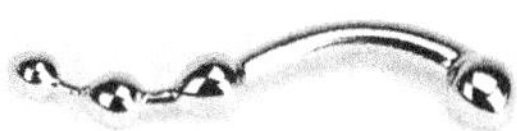

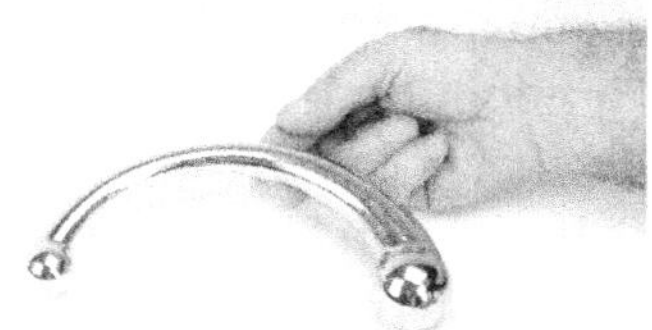

N-Joy™ produces two products that I think you'll find absolutely delightful. They are the Fun Wand® and the Pure Wand®.

1. The dual-purpose Fun Wand® is, in my opinion, the best dildo I've ever used on a woman. Made of surgical steel and nicely thin, the woman doesn't have to be concerned about *width* as you start to play sexually. I am particularly fond of this toy and recommend it highly. I suspect that you'll find that the side with the three balls elicits squeal after squeal as they move in and out of your lady's vaginal opening; the side with the single large rounded end makes an excellent G-spot manipulator.

2. The Pure Wand®, with one much larger end, is even better as a G-spot manipulator. Frankly, I'd recommend both to you. For the ladies, it's either a G-spot pleaser or an anal toy. For the guys, it's a prostate massager.

Fork You™

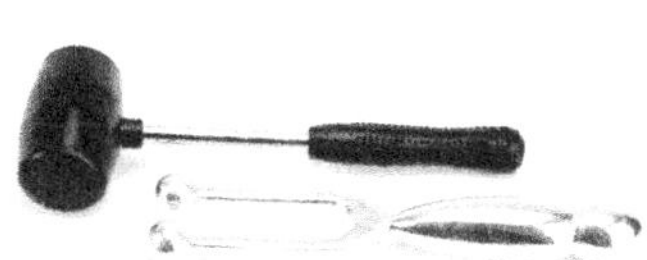

I'm going to include this dildo, although it is not in production right now. I'm including it to show you an example of a very creative dildo — because new and interesting items come on the market fairly often. This curiosity was designed by Tristan Taormino (author of The Ultimate Guide to Anal Sex for Women) who now has some other interesting dildos listed on her website. This dildo, though is a one-piece stainless steel item with a tuning fork on the opposite end. You insert it and strike the tuning fork end with a rubber mallet that you keep around for this solitary purpose. If you're into anal play, of course, it's just the thing.

By the way, if you *are* able to find one, a word of caution: when you hit it with the mallet, be sure to have a finger under the neck where the tuning fork tines come together into a short shaft before connecting with the body of the toy. You have to place your finger there in order to stabilize it. If you don't stabilize it, when you bonk it, it will suddenly jerk upwards inside your lady and somewhat ruin both her mood and her estimation of your mastery over this toy. The fact that you say something like, "Oops, sorry," is not likely to improve matters. And giggling at her reaction is *certainly* likely to put a stop to further play. (Yes — unfortunately, you're listening to personal experiences, here.)

Glass Dildos

[Note: This section is adapted and presented here, with permission, from an article by Anne Bryne that appeared in the premier issue of Power Exchange Magazine, January 2007. She also provided the samples used to make these photos.]

For several years, glass sex toys have been featured on HBO's "Real Sex," and in *Playboy, Penthouse,* and *Hustler* Magazines. They are widely available both online and in retail stores. As prices can range from about $30.00 to over $400.00, it raises the question, "What's going on, here?"

Because the glass sex toys can be made to incorporate bumps and swirls that can provide a different range of sensations than silicone or rubber dildos, and because glass sex toys can be extremely artistically appealing, glass dildos are often attractive for ladies. If you're just starting out with glass dildos, probes or wand shapes are probably the best choices, as they often have a ball at each end that can provide varied sensations. These probes or wands come in many colors, weights, and textures. It is often possible to mix three types of sensations with one glass object — the smoothness of the glass itself, textured ribbing, and bumps that can accentuate both in-and-out motion and also G-spot stimulation.

Glass Basics

1. ***Built to Last a Lifetime:*** Unless you drop it on a hard surface, these things are nearly indestructible.

2. ***Easy to Heat or to Cool:*** Glass holds heat/cold very well, but you must ALWAYS test their temperature before use. Heating or cooling a glass toy is a fairly slow process that must be planned; you should allow approximately 30 minutes for heating or cooling your glass sex toy.

    a. Never microwave the glass; it could explode. Instead, submerge your glass in warm tap water for about five minutes. Pour off about two thirds of the water and replace that amount with hotter water and let stand for 15 – 20 minutes, depending on the size of the toy. Be sure you have determined the temperature of the water by inserting a meat thermometer into the water bowl.

    b. To cool your glass sex toy, never freeze it; it could shatter when inserted into a person who is 98-degrees. Equally serious, it could freeze itself onto her skin. Simply fill a pan with cool water, wait 5 minutes and — if you're particularly sadistic — add a couple of ice cubes. Note: She's not likely to like this, and it may ruin your seductive evening. Being clever with temperature play is not a good idea unless you've pre-negotiated it.

Safety Warning #7: Your lady's body temperature is about 98-degrees. Heat much over 105-degrees or coolness much below room temperature is going to be quite a shock. Do not waiver from these temperature guidelines unless you're used to temperature play and have pre-negotiated this with the lady. Failure to follow these suggestions will likely produce an unhappy sex partner — or worse.

> **Safety Warning Continued:** In the "worse" category, Jay Wiseman, an attorney with years and years of experience as an EMT, added this comment: "There is a BIG point here: Sudden exposure to severe cold, particularly in the vagina or anus, can produce a vagal-mediated reflex that can slow the heartbeat. Every, now and then, the heartbeat can be slowed down to *zero*. In other words, there is a potential for the use of extremely cold items to cause cardiac arrest. This risk is likely elevated in 'older' ladies — whatever 'older' means."

3. ***Easy to Clean and Sterilize:*** You should wipe the glass down with either of the previously-mentioned medical wipes. Failing that, at least run them through your dishwasher with the drying heat-cycle turned on. Be aware, though, that since your dishwasher is not a medical autoclave, you're not *really* sterilizing them, so you would need to sanitize them.

4. ***Won't Transfer Body Fluids:*** As glass is non-porous, it absorbs nothing. That means that once you've disinfected them, you can use them with other sex partners without any concern about transfer of body fluids. Also, because glass is non-porous, it is odor resistant.

5. ***Erotic Art:*** Unlike other working sex toys, many of these objects are works of art that are visually stimulating and easily displayed without calling attention to their erotic use. I have a friend who uses this toy on her formal dinning room table as a knife rest. She mentioned to me that several of her friends have commented on her "Lovely example of Depression-Era glass." She simply smiled.

6. ***Variety:*** Glass sex toys come in a wide and growing array of shapes, colors and sizes: ranging from *spinners, juicers, rotary,* or *G-spot,* all the way to foot-long *batons*. As they are highly individualized, you'll want to see and feel any glass you intend to add to your collection,

Kinds of Glass Sex Toys

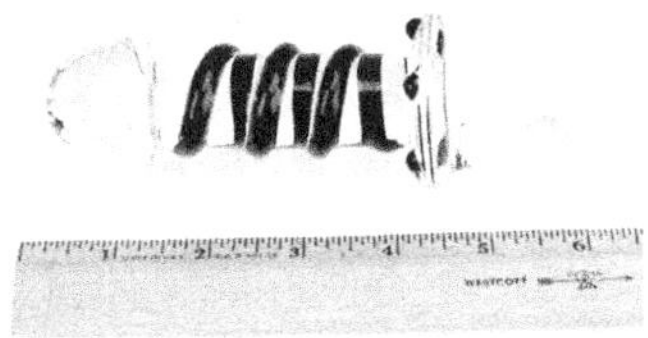

Spinners, Juicers, and Rotary Glass Sex Toys: These terms describe glass sex toys that are made with a handle. Often, they have either a smooth penile shaped head, or an egg-shaped head for ease of entry. Look for glass that is one-piece, rather than glass made from joining two separate pieces. Often these toys will include both ribbing around the shaft and bumps on the shaft (if it has bumps, it's sometimes referred to as "Huck glass"). This is a glass toy that will give you an opportunity to provide several different sensations. Spinners or juicers generally have an insertable length of approximately 3½ inches and are used either for anal or for vaginal use. Of the glass toys, this is one of my favorites; ladies often squeal through the twisting sensations.

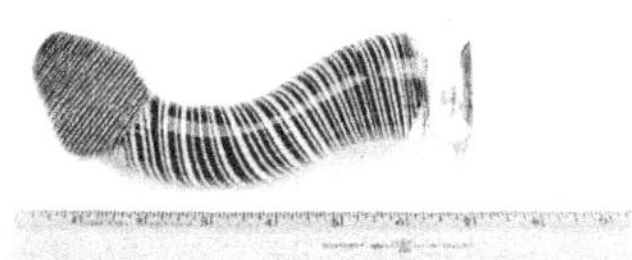

G-spot Glass Sex Toys: This is a term used to describe any number of glass sex toys that have a bend in them specifically designed to stimulate the female G-spot. These toys come in an astounding variety of shapes, colors, variations, weights, lengths, and prices. Here, you can find something for every aesthetic taste.

While originally designed to target the G-spot, these styles have evolved into a large variety of curved shapes that have many uses. For example, they are now finding their way into use as prostate stimulators. They can be smooth with beautiful patterns encased on the inside, or wrapped in beautiful dichroic (two-colored) glass. If you are looking at a wrapped piece, make sure that you are buying a dichroic wrapping, not a spray-painted covering of color. This will ensure that the lovely intense colors will remain on your piece during use, and not remain within your lover.

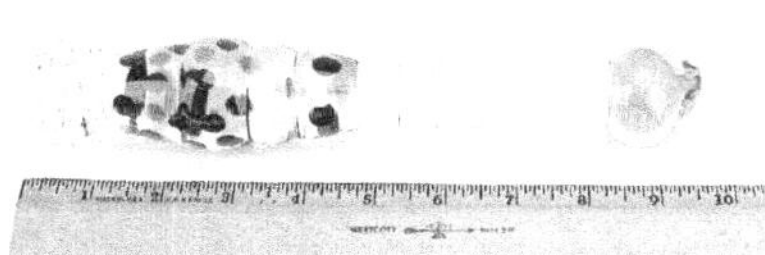

Batons with Handles: Glass dildos with handles, also known as *love batons*, are glass sex toys that work well either solo or with a partner. The handle provides a nice grip, and enables you to work it just the way you (or your partner) prefer. These are also often considered (and sometimes labeled) *extreme* on some sites, due to their

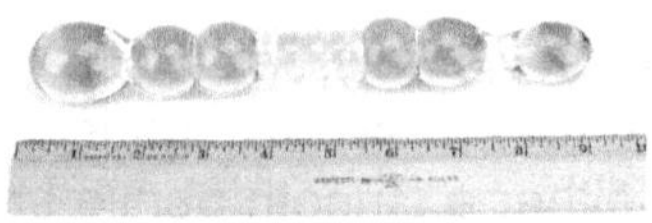

larger, longer size. With these toys, you need to take care that you don't insert them further than is comfortable for your playmate. In some cases, it is possible for two women to play with these toys at one time. I like these glass sex toys because they provide two, three, or four different sensations in one instrument. I find them well received.

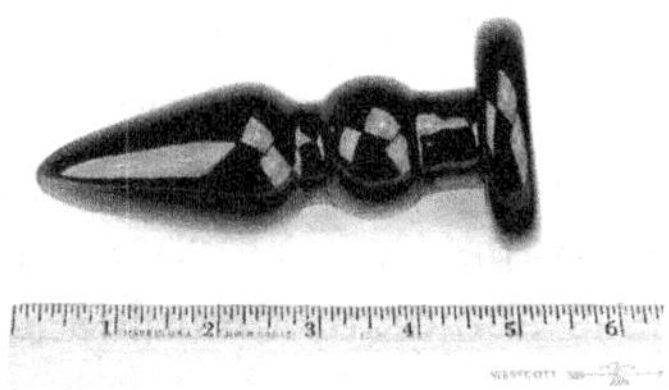

Anal Probe, Anal Butt Plugs: These glass sex toys are shorter, and are generally flared at the base. A plug will usually have a flat base in order that the user may sit down with the plug in place. Plugs will have either an egg head, or more commonly, a pointed head. These are shaped this way to facilitate entry.

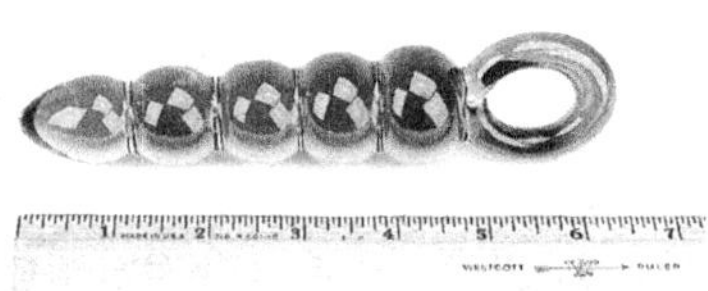

A *probe* may appear much like a smaller version of a *baton* or possibly a glass *G-spot Wand*. To differentiate, look for a ball head for anal ease of entry with some type of shaft, ripples, balls (sometimes called a "popper") with a lollipop handle. All of these can provide wonderful new sensations.

It's Not Quite Glass, But...

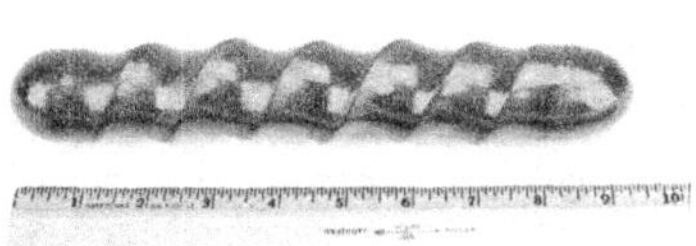

A new line of granite dildos is making its debut in this country. Both masculine and erotic, I personally find these extremely appealing.

Specialty Dildos

The Accommodator®

Well, it's certainly a dildo, but unless you have a bulletproof personal reputation and are very secure in your masculinity, you probably don't want to try this one in public. A woman highly recommended the *Accommodator®* to me. It combines dildo functions with cunnilingus activity. While it looks silly, it wins a woman's heart in large part simply because you are willing to put the thing on to please her. It costs about $25 and, like the others, is also carried by many sex toy stores.

Now for a dose of reality: You may find that some women can't take the entire length of this item, especially until they become sexually excited and their vaginal canals lengthen. So, there you are, with this protrusion sticking into her and you can't *quite* reach her vulva (let alone her clitoris) with your tongue. However, this approach may win her heart by demonstrating how willing you are to look silly for her. Up to you, of course. Try an Internet search for *The Accommodator*.

By the way, you can accomplish about as much sensation by inserting a nice dildo while licking.

Inflatable Dildos

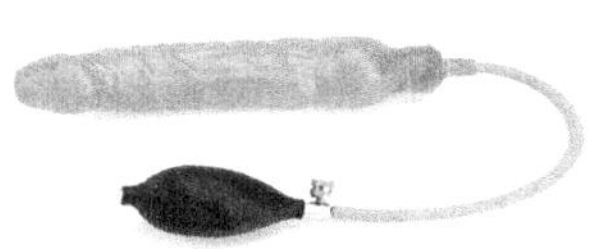

This toy is great for building up to fisting. They are widely available either in sex stores or on the Internet. You can use it in conjunction with the next entry — what I affectionately call my Outrageously Huge Dildo. Here, the progression is to start with fingering, move up to a larger dildo, move up to the inflatable unit, and then insert the outrageously huge dildo. After that, it's going to be your latex-gloved fist — with lots and lots of water-based lube. (Some years ago, when I bought what I now simply call the "larger dildo," my wife took one look at it and said, "You must be joking." It's interesting how perspectives change over the years. Now, that toy is used as a good starting point with some ladies.)

Outrageously HUGE

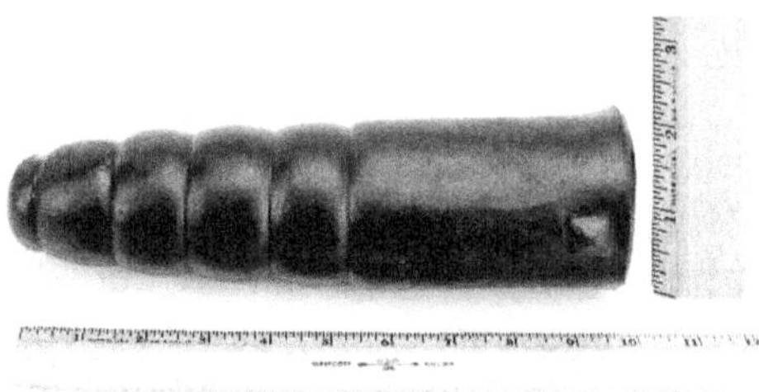

Dildos of this type are great for building up to fisting (not their intended purpose, but that's another story). But you'd better talk about this guy before you get too far into your evening. They come larger than this one — quite a bit larger, in fact — but I've never encountered a lady for whom this was not large enough. You're most likely to find these in stores or Internet sites that cater to gay sex toys.

When not in use and left casually on your bedside table, they can serve double-duty as mindfuck decoration for Visiting Ladies. But be careful; unless you're playing with an adventurous lady, you may ruin the mood-du-jour by terrorizing her. Brought out casually and presented to her as the next dildo to be used, you may find that the next phrase that passes your lips — as she's dressing to leave — is, "Well, may I call you tomorrow?" You know you've made a really serious tactical error when she turns to scowl at you as she stomps out.

Chapter Summary

This brief chapter was devoted to a review of some of my most favorite dildos. I discussed steel dildos, glass dildos, and specialty dildos. In many cases, I explained why I liked that kind of dildo, and how you might consider using it.

Part IV

Lights, Camera, Action

Chapter Eight

Erotic Shaving

Many men and women prefer that their partners shave their genital regions. For many — myself included — a shaved lady is extremely erotic (a fetish, actually). However, many women won't consider being shaved, so you'd better check with your sexual partner to determine her level of interest in being clean-shaven down there.

For men, removing their own pubic hair can make the area around their penises seem more sensitive and also make their penises appear much larger — a turn-on for some women. (Out of curiosity, I recently asked a family practice physician friend of mine to estimate the number of men who shaved their privates. To my surprise, he said that in his experience, about 20% to 30% of his patients shaved.)

Erotic shaving comes in two flavors: safety razors and straightedge razors.

1. If you're going to be using a **safety** razor, then buy a 3-blade or 4-blade model. Please avoid the single-blade disposable razors; they're much more likely to nick your lady — the result then being a less-than-stellar shaving session. Even if you're using a safety razor for her shave, I do encourage you to get an old-fashioned bristled shaving brush and shaving mug to add to the ceremony. They're inexpensive, and they look great. Don't lose sight of the fact that an erotic shaving session is about mood and setting, not about getting it done quickly.

I didn't list the shaving brush or shaving mug below, as they are optional. If you purchase these, then put some of the gel in the shaving cup, dilute with a little bit of warm water and apply with the shaving brush.

2. **Straightedge** shaving is an art form. Because it can be so dangerous and because this is a skill that is best taught one-on-one, I will not address it in this book.

Starting Out

Lay Out Your Equipment

1. Set up a massage table or a well-padded (and very sturdy) dining room table. I don't recommend a bed, as beds are a bit too low.

2. Cover the massage table with a sheet and provide a pillow.

3. Cover the sheet with a nice oversized bath or beach towel.

4. Place a small bath towel under the area on which the woman's backside will be positioned. This smaller towel is used to catch water dripping between her legs or down her sides. Avoid soaking the large bath or beach towel; sitting on a cold, wet towel after the shave will be a mood-breaker. Your lady is not likely to think that sitting on a cold, wet towel is very sexy.

5. Provide a bowl of warm/hot water containing a washcloth. If you are going to be doing this frequently, I highly recommend a 4-cup soup warmer. It has a thermostatic control on it and warms up almost immediately.

6. Place a dry hand towel (used to dry the woman after shaving) in front of the bowl of water.

7. Place a coffee cup (or equivalent) filled with warm water (used for rinsing hairs off the razor) near the larger container of warm/hot water.

8. Place the shaving gel next to the little cup of warm water. It is my strong recommendation that you use a gel, and not soap. And select a hypoallergenic gel for sensitive skin. You want hypoallergenic gel, because it will produce a close shave without leaving little red bumps.

9. Place the razor next to the shaving gel. As previously mentioned, I recommend that you use a safety razor that has two, three, or four blades. You might even consider giving the razor to the lady as a memento of the occasion.

> **Safety Warning #8:** I strongly recommend that you not use disposable razors; they are likely to nick and cut the lady. Always use a new blade each time you're going to be doing a genital shave. Unless you're fluid bonded, once the blade has been used, discard it immediately.

10. You will benefit from using clippers, scissors, or barber's shears prior to using the razor if the woman is presently unshaven.

11. Don't forget to include an extension cord in your pre-planning checklist, if electrical shears are involved, or if you intend to use electric-powered vibrators after the shaving scene (in which case you also need to set out the vibrators you may want to use).

12. Select your sensual music.

Almost Ready

1. Be sure the room isn't too cold for a naked lady

2. Turn on the sensual music

3. Light the candles

4. Turn down the room lights

5. Be sure the washcloth that is in the warm/hot water is not too hot

6. To get in the mood, the two of you may wish to take a very long, warm bath beforehand. If your bathtub won't fit two people, at least propose a shower for her. This is not only part of mood-setting, but also the warm water helps to prepare her skin for the upcoming shave. (This stage is optional.)

The Shave

1. Ask your lady to come to the shaving area and lie down on the massage table or alternative. Place most of the small shaving items between your partner's legs or nearby on a side table.

2. If your subject has long pubic hairs, trim her hair with electric clippers or scissors before you begin using a razor or you'll clog the blade with the first cut of about half-an-inch.

3. Take the washcloth that is in the hot water, squeeze it dry, place it over the area to be shaved, and massage gently. (You've seen this in movies — a barber puts a hot towel on a man's face before an old-fashioned straightedge shave.) Right about now, a vibrator of her choice feels really nice. Don't overdo the vibrator at this stage; orgasm isn't the goal; shaving is the goal.

4. Apply shaving cream (or gel) a few minutes before shaving to soften hairs. Consider using a shaving cream with additional conditioners, anti-bacterial agents or aloe, so long as she has no allergies to these products. As you'll read in Taw Preston's book, he uses Noxzema® cream as the shaving lotion. He also uses alum on the thumb of the hand not holding the razor (available in the condiments section of most grocery stores) to stretch the woman's skin tight to help get a close shave. Alum provides the grip you'll need when your lady has wet skin.

5. Be sure to use a new replaceable blade.

6. When shaving, try not to stroke an area more than twice; you don't want to create a skin irritation. On the first stroke, stroke with the grain (the direction the hair is growing) to remove most of the hair, then stroke against the grain for a smooth, close shave. If the *against* stroke irritates your partner, then skip that and use both strokes with the grain. For some people, shaving the pubic area against the grain can lead to painful ingrown hairs. As you become more experienced with genital shaving, you may be able to take more than two strokes in an area. Please remember: If this is a first-time event, be as conservative as you can be; the goal is to relax your lady and give her a good experience. The first few times you do this, a good experience is better than a perfect shave.

7. Once the shave is over, use your warm water source to rinse the washcloth. Clean soap from the area. Before you dry her off, consider again placing the hot washcloth (squeezed dry) over the entire area. This is very relaxing. Then, pat her dry with the fresh bath towel substitute. If you want to add a touch of real elegance, consider pre-warming the towel. I recommend that you leave the dry towel in place while you gently apply her chosen vibrator to extract a sigh of relaxation from her lips. But no, you are not to bring her to orgasm, yet.

A Few Warnings

1. Some people have allergic reactions to some shaving creams. The pubic area is often quite sensitive. If your newly shaved partner develops a reaction, natural perspiration and abrasion from clothing may make this area uncomfortable for a few days. If this happens — despite using hypoallergenic shaving gel — consider removing erotic shaving from your play repertoire.
2. Letting hair grow out after shaving your pubic area is a bitch. The sharp hairs —combined with the sensitive skin — will make you realize just how much movement happens in that area on an average day. Chaffing is nearly unavoidable. Message: Once you start shaving her pubic area, she will want either to continue the practice or firmly discontinue the practice.
3. **DO NOT USE POWDER.** If you must use a powder, please use cornstarch. Powder contains talc, which has been linked directly with ovarian cancer.

In conclusion, you should speak with your partner about arranging to shave one another. This can be a very erotic, sensual activity. Be sure to communicate clearly during the shaving scene and proceed slowly and lovingly. Work to discern what your partner likes. Ask her what does and does not feel good.

If you find you love the soft feel of her shaved genitals, consider commercial waxing. While you can purchase the commercial supplies to do this yourself, I've not had much success with that. NOTE: If your lady tends to get ingrown hairs, waxing may not be for her.

If the two of you really fall in love with the shaved feel, but she is less interested in shaving every day, you might consider treating your lady to the gift of a multi-treatment laser hair-removal process. They run upwards of $1,500, but she'll never shave again. (Note: Laser hair removal seems not to work the same on all colors of hair. Be sure to do some research to verify your lady's hair is a good candidate for this process.)

Chapter Summary

This chapter on erotic shaving guided you from equipment setup to drying her off after the shave was completed. Along the way, I discussed some safety warnings as well as the techniques that should enable you to deliver a lovely shaving experience to your lady.

Chapter Nine

The Art and Science of Oral Sex with Women

First, for those just dying to know, the word *cunnilingus* comes from the joining of two Latin words. First, the alternative Latin word for the vulva (cunnus) added to the Latin word for tongue (lingua). Those who research this field note that while most women can orgasm from clitoral stimulation, only about one-third of women orgasm easily during the actual act of intercourse. Which is why you're going to want to consider becoming an expert in this area.

In order not to overwhelm you by combining both cunnilingus and fingering techniques in one chapter, I'm starting with oral sex and reserving the next chapter for fingering techniques. Yes, they're used together after she's warmed up, but you're going to have to decide when to initiate the fingering and when to go back to licking. That is, you're in charge of designing and pacing the sexual play. It's rather like *leading* in a dance. The leader (usually the man) has to figure out the next sequence of moves based upon the lady's skill level. In this case, your pacing of oral and fingering techniques is determined by the woman's reactions and responses. We're back to the underlying theme of this book: monitor your lady's reactions and ask for feedback until she confirms that you've become very good at reading her reactions to your actions.

Personal Note #4: When I start to play with a new lady, it usually takes me about half-a-dozen times with her before I feel comfortable that I know what she wants. First encounters, while always exciting, are seldom magical. The more encounters we have, the longer the sexual play sessions grow, and the more interested she becomes in our next sexual play session.

Opening Statement: It will transform your sex life (and stand you apart from most lovers) once you become a master at pleasing a woman orally. In many cases, providing excellent service in this area affects how she is going to treat you later in the evening. This being so, here are some hints, tips, and suggestions.

You've heard me say this one over and over: The secret to pleasing your lady with tongue, lips, chin, and nose is to ask her whether she likes this or that, read her signs of satisfaction (or dissatisfaction), and modify your actions in response. You could be the best sexual mechanic in the world, but if you can't read your partner's emotional road signs, you're going to end up wandering around in a desolate labial wasteland until you eventually drop from exhaustion or get fired. All this will happen without having provided her the cherished orgasm.

Tip #16: Cunnilingus may produce a recurring "ohmygodohmygod" reaction in your woman throughout your sexual play. If she's not physically or orally expressing her pleasure at your actions, you might want to check in to be certain that what you're doing is what she wants done. In the alternative, you may be playing with a lady who is not very expressive. It's up to you to discover which it is. Again, ask questions.

Things You Must Know Before You Play Sexually

There's a Chinese proverb that says that if you save a person's life, they're yours forever. I think you'll find that if you can deliver hair-pulling, nail-sinking, screaming orgasms using your sexual techniques, you'll have won yourself a sex partner for as long as you wish.

Don't Be Confused

Some men think that oral sex is just a way to make her wet down there so they can start intercourse. Not meaning to offend anyone, I would like you to consider that that's not it. Cunnilingus is the meal and intercourse is dessert — at least for many, many women.

Although admittedly sampling a small sub-population of all women, The Janus Report on Sexual Behavior by Samuel S. and Cynthia L. Janus reports that "...a whopping 92% of 'career women' surveyed prefer oral sex to any other sex act." In this light, guys are highly advised to master this form of sexual play. And remember, unless your lady is really, really used to cunnilingus, she may have some barriers to overcome. US advertising culture makes women think that they're smelly and require all sorts of douches, deodorants, and powders (very dangerous, this) in order to be presentable. You're soon going to run into ladies who will be astonished that vibrators, cunnilingus, and fingering are some of your favorite sexual activities, and that you aren't in this just to satisfy yourself. I think you're going to find that very few of their previous partners really seemed to enjoy it — they merely tolerated it in order to gain sexual access.

Be Sure You're Both Psychologically Prepared

First, don't try to go down on your lady unless you're in the mood; performing cunnilingus when you don't want to is likely to show. A good cunnilingus session is likely to give her a renewed rosy picture of you. To help prepare yourself for your evening:

- Shower
- Dress up in something special
- Relax and unwind
- Discuss your intentions and get her feedback and permission

Second, be prepared to be very sensitive to any unease on your lady's part.

Some women who receive oral sex feel emotionally exposed. This is particularly true of dominant ladies; they may feel that cunnilingus requires them to surrender too much control to the man, and they won't permit that. Related to that comment, one lady said that while she didn't feel that the man pleasing her orally was necessarily dominating her, that when she gave oral pleasure to a man, she definitely felt in control and actually preferred giving to receiving in this area.

Another woman commented that she was turned off to receiving oral sex when she was married to a man who didn't know what he was doing and wouldn't follow suggestions to make oral sex feel better. Worse, he acted "put out" with the situation. She went on to comment that, "I'm willing to bet — and in fact think — that women who don't like receiving oral sex has more to do with 'Not being comfortable with their sexuality' or with 'men who don't bother to become familiar with the correct technique or how a woman's body works.'" She went on to note, too, that many women have religious taboos to overcome when cunnilingus is involved.

Couple the emotional exposure with the reality that cunnilingus requires physical exposure, and you can understand why some women may be less enthusiastic about the activity than you had expected. Certainly, not every woman is going to feel vulnerable with your face between her legs. Indeed, some will be empowered and others are just going to feel that they are being really well-pleased. My point is that you need to be particularly sensitive to the woman's psychological reaction to your advances and activities.

Now, while we're on the topic of your being sensitive to her feelings and getting feedback before you begin this activity, let me summarize a true story. This is a landmine story.

This lady had been sexually abused as a child. After years of work, she had put these experiences behind her when she was raped by a drug addict who pinned her down and engaged in cunnilingus. Many years later, after she thought this issue was completely flattened, a male friend she had been getting to know apparently decided that he had "passed inspection" and was so pleased, that he spontaneously decided to reward her with a session of oral sex. A combination of his sudden movement, plus the shock of a particular sensation, caused her to have a flashback. She now comments:

> "If he had started out by asking me how I felt about oral sex, he would have known about this background and would have been more sensitive. He might have even rewarded me in another way. But, by starting to make advances without warning, my body reacted before my mind could... that kind of fear is NOT fun."

While oral sex can be a landmine for some, other women may avoid oral sex for almost the opposite reason. One lady I know once told me that she avoids it because the sensations are so intense; she's scared that she'll kick the guy as she thrashes around.

In a similar vein, one late-20s lady said quite firmly that to receive cunnilingus, she has to be passive and she simply isn't interested in being passive during sex.

So, discuss your oral sex ideas with your lady before your evening begins. Tell her what you have in mind and listen sensitively to her comments. Also, realize that you're taking the most delicate, vulnerable part of your lover's body — her genitals — and placing them between the most potentially vicious, animalistic part of yours — your teeth. That's bound to give her pause at some level of consciousness.

Now, if all of this is not enough, some women are prone to the *Four Fears*. You need to know them and be prepared to overcome them.

- ***I'm anxious about getting undressed in front of you:*** I'm not comfortable with my body. Some women aren't happy with their shape. They're likely to be tense when it comes to getting undressed out of fear that you'll say something — and they've built up hopes and expectations about this encounter. They may be thinking, "I'm overweight and my clothes don't fit me properly." In the first place, despite the well-known American cultural fixation with Barbie-like figures, not all men are interested in that. Also, some men aren't particularly sensitive to the lady's physical shape. Now, it may even be that you aren't thrilled with your own shape. But men — much more than women — take their bodies rather as a fact of life. So, this is where you need to be reassuring, kind, and very, very careful. Chapter 11 covers this general area in detail.

- ***I'm not pretty down there:*** I don't look normal down there; my inner lips are too small/too large. My clitoris is too small/too large. The trouble with this thought is that most men are likely to be fairly oblivious to the shape of their lady's vulva, inner lips, or the size of her clitoris.

- ***I'll take too long to orgasm:*** What's the hurry? Can you think of another way to have more fun for a couple of hours?

- ***I might smell and/or taste bad:*** This topic is so sensitive that I want to discuss it in some detail right now.

Odor and Taste

As this area is so emotionally loaded, I'd like to address it head-on in this subsection. The odor and taste of a woman can be divided into two very separate categories: Odor as a result of infection or uncleanness, and odor as a function of body chemistry.

Infection or Uncleanness: If your lady is emitting a strong odor from her vagina, she may have an infection. Infections can occur for several reasons: vaginal bacterial overgrowth, sexually transmitted infections (STIs), or from wearing tight or damp clothing, particularly those made of synthetic material (e.g., nylon pantyhose). In the case of the nylon pantyhose, they may not allow sufficient air flow to the area around the vulva. Alternatively, your lady may have an odor that has resulted from eating certain foods or from excessive sweating.

As your lady's odor is going to be a delicate subject to bring up, you might want to go to the website www.goaskalice.columbia.edu for suggestions. In addition to the quote below, she provides a wealth of useful information on sexual topics. At any rate, her suggestion about odor is to use some phrasing like this, "I want to mention something that is hard to talk about. I really like you, and I enjoy getting to know your body and giving you pleasure. I know that every woman has her own scent, and since I'm becoming more familiar with your body, I'm wondering if this is your usual smell. I've noticed that it's strong, and I'm having trouble getting used to it."

Yeast infections, a fairly common event for women, will not only change her odor, but will cause her to produce more copious amounts of white, creamy discharge than at times when she does not have a yeast infection. Also, if you're thinking of ungloved vaginal fisting, you have a greater likelihood of introducing bacteria that may cause her to get a case of *bacterial vaginosis* — or some other infection — from your dirty fingernails. If that happens, then she **will** have an odor. This odor is quite distinctive; it smells like decaying fish. Worse, to get rid of it, she's likely to have to take a trip to her gynecologist and then take a course of antibiotics specific to the problem. This, then, adds a substantial cost to that lovely ungloved fingering or fisting session.

Moral: If you are going to put your fingers into your lady, take extra care to thoroughly clean your hands and scrub under your fingernails. Ideally, you should wear either latex (or latex-free) gloves. By the way, I've had more than one lady comment that she vastly prefers that a man wear gloves and add lube; that the slick, slippery feeling is *much* better than she gets from an ungloved hand with lube.

> **Safety Warning #9:** Some people are allergic to latex. This affects their ability to put latex on their hands or penis, and it also affects what the man can wear to touch a lady with such allergies. If this is an issue for you, try an Internet search for topics such as non-latex gloves or non-latex condoms.

Body chemistry: In chemistry, the pH range runs from 0 (strong acid) to 14 (strong base). Skin has a pH of 6-7 — practically neutral. A vagina's pH is in the 3.8-4.5 range, something like red wine, and the pH of coffee is about 5.0; the pH of sperm is about 8.

This means that she's going to be *tart* when you first start playing. As the woman warms up sexually, her pH will rise and become more neutral; this means not only that her vagina becomes less pungent, but also that it becomes more hospitable for sperm. However, once you've ejaculated inside your lady, for the lady to avoid emitting a strong odor, the semen left in the vagina needs to be removed fairly soon. This is because semen (a protein) has a pH of about 8 and will be acted upon chemically as the woman's pH starts heading back toward its unaroused rate of the 3.8 – 4.5 range.

My final note involving pH is this: Soap has a pH from 7-14. This will be **very** upsetting to an ecosystem that prefers a pH of about 4.0. Related to this, douching has earned a bad reputation because it can cause serious trauma to the good bacteria that live in your lady's vagina. Please do not encourage douching unless there is an unpleasant odor. "Douching is extremely harsh and is one of the biggest causes of vaginal infections." Ultimate Guide to Cunnilingus p. 70. A persistent foul odor is cause to visit the doctor.

Be Physically Prepared for Intercourse

You may need to take an erection enhancer of your choice, either prescription or herbal. As there are many options, you're going to have to do some research of your own. You might start by consulting your physician. Both for prescription and non-prescription approaches, you're going to have to experiment to find one (or a combination) that works for you. I've used a few herbals with great success, then recommended them to other guys who've had a range of reactions, from nothing to fabulous. Note: If you have high blood pressure or are on medications to lower your blood pressure, the treatment of erectile dysfunction becomes more complex and absolutely requires that you follow your physician's recommendations.

And you're going to have to exercise — particularly if you're still engaging in intercourse. Unless you can comfortably sustain an elevated pulse for many minutes, you may have trouble delivering the kind of sexual performance most women seek.

Some Tips and Techniques

Be Sure to Negotiate Touch and No Touch Zones

Although the issue of negotiation is threaded throughout this book, I want to bring it up now because this issue can sneak up on you at times and leave you confused by your lady's reaction to something you thought was a non-issue. To make this particularly graphic, I'll tell you a true story. One time, as I was negotiating sex play with a lovely lady, she started out by quite firmly stating that if I touched her belly button, she'd get up and leave. Okay, message received. However, she went on to say, toe-sucking was definitely in. Got it. I'm in. Let's go.

> **Tip #17:** It's important to discuss with your lady what you're planning for your evening's sexual play. Nobody likes uncomfortable surprises; they can kill the evening or the relationship.

Learn How to Kiss

Every so often, *kissing* comes up in conversations with ladies. I know a number of very experienced ladies who absolutely positively will not let you play with them unless they like the way you kiss. The *Kama Sutra* identifies 14 ways of kissing. The Marcy Michaels book Going Down gives lots of very specific kissing advice and technique coaching. For starters, try coming present the next time you kiss for passion. Revel in what it is you're doing. My God, you have a woman to have sex with! Communicate how special that is for you. (Yes, even if you've been married 35 years.)

Be Sure She's Wet

If you start playing and you find that her inner lips and/or vagina are dry, go back to kissing and caressing for a while. Once you're sure the lady is lubricated, you can advance your sexual play. There's nothing worse than rushing into this, so make sure she's really turned on before you get down to serious sex.

> **Tip #18:** Don't head straight for her clit: I highly recommend that you start all cunnilingus sessions with indirect stimulation. Her clitoris is only part of the story you're telling with your tongue and your fingers. You're going for teasing here, not conquest. And you should have been kissing and nibbling all over her body as you undressed her — unless you **tore** her clothes off ("Another topic for pre-negotiation?" I asked. "No," he sighed, "I'll just replace them.")

Learn Where to Touch

The major erogenous zones are as follows:

- Ears, both front and back
- Nape of neck
- Lips
- Under arms
- Inside of elbow
- Inside of wrists
- Fingers (that you insert into your mouth and suck on slowly)
- Breasts
- Tummy

- Inside of knee
- Feet/toes

In other words, you can pretty much turn her whole body into an erogenous zone. It's all in your approach.

I think you'll be in for a really pleasant surprise at your lady's reaction when she is in a highly aroused state, and you stretch her arm away from her body, palm up, and lick the inside of her elbow, and then lick the inside of her wrist. Still on the wrist, you might consider adding some spice by growling with a low, deep growl, and then sink your teeth into her wrist (no, you don't actually bite her; shame on you). If she bathed before you started, consider asking her not to put on any deodorant; you'll want to be able to lick her underarms without coming up with a mouthful of deodorant. Seriously icky. You'd be surprised at the number of ladies who think that underarm licking is a *huge* turn-on (well, at least *I* was surprised). Expect serious thrashing and delighted screaming the first time you try this with a lady; be sure you have her reasonably pinned to the bed. Remember, you're supposed to be *playing*.

Learn How to Touch

Don't start by sticking your fingers in her vagina. And, even after you have her somewhat aroused, don't play your trump card too soon by putting your fingers all the way inside. In the first place, someone is likely to visit you and demand that you surrender your *Great Lover* ID card. In the second place, these actions will certainly detract from the upcoming penetration and kill the tease factor. Try to remember that much of a woman's pleasure is about yearning. Moving too soon is sure to dampen the fire of her fantasies. And when you start to enter her with your fingers, try starting out by inserting one finger only about a half-an-inch to an inch. Then insert a second finger to the same depth, then go in about half an inch more. Then come out. Anyway, we'll cover this a bit later under "fingering techniques."

Consider Options About Physical Positions During Cunnilingus

There are advantages and disadvantages of each of the positions I'm about to name. They're here for your review so that we're all on the same page. These certainly are not in any kind of order-of-importance.

Woman on her back (these three positions are good if you are going to bite or grab on to an outer lip):

- You're on your knees along side of your lady, facing south. This way, she can fondle your penis and scrotum, if she's so inclined.
- You've flattened out from that kneeling position and are now lying next to her. Your body alignment is about the same as above; your rear end is about even with her head and you're along side her with your head between her legs. Now, she cannot get sexual access to you. You may want to use this to limit her distractions while you're pleasuring her.
- You're lying between her open legs; your feet are probably dangling over the edge of the bed. Clearly, this position stops her ability to get anywhere near your genital area, but you now have a birds-eye view (so to speak), and can lick, finger, or use most of your toys on her while she simply concentrates on the sensations that you are providing.

Woman on her knees, you approaching from behind.

- When she tilts her rear end upwards, this gives access both to her vaginal area and to her anus, for those of you who desire it. Licking from this position often flows rather quickly into intercourse. It also is a great position for using dildos and vibrators.

One action, various combinations of positions

- You're parallel with her, on top of her, beside her, or under her — in the well-known "69" position. Unless your lady likes what she can do to you in this position, you're rather squashing her, if you're on top.

Oral Technique — Phase One of Sex Play

Pre-touch/lick Commentaries

If you find that cunnilingus is tiring to you, you may not be resting your tongue correctly in your mouth. This will affect many things related to oral sex, including your ability to perform for a long time. Please refer to the Michaels book listed in Appendix A: Start at page six for a discussion of your tongue's correct placement in your mouth. As she points out, a quick check of your tongue control can be made with a common breakfast cereal. Try to swallow while you hold bit of cereal against the roof of your mouth with the tip of your tongue (see her chapter ten).

Develop Your Technique: Once she's starting to show excitement, it's time to start licking. Get your fingers out of there and don't touch anything for a bit. Consider your range of options. Start by kissing around her breasts and stomach and slowly working your way down. You might consider licking and nibbling the underside of her breasts — it's an area that is seldom addressed and that is highly sensitive. Unless you absolutely know that she likes the amount of attention you're paying to her breasts, don't get carried away with fondling them; it's too cliché. Anyway, right now it's all about the stomach and inner thighs. A little bit of licking interspersed with *gentle* biting is good, but a sure winner is to start at her knee and move towards her private parts in a slow, shark-like swoop. But *skip over her vulva* and pick another lick/bite area. Remember, you're trying to prolong the foreplay and build sexual tension.

Mons Play: At some point in your activities, you'll want to push down on her mons with firm (but not hard) pressure. If done correctly, this should result in an engorgement of blood throughout her genital area. This, in turn, leads to greater sensitivity — a good thing.

Add Some Heat: This is a good time to consider adding some heat-producing genital stimulant cream — previously discussed. You'll find that a generous application both outside and inside the lady's vagina will bring a smile to her lips. Be sure that the cream is recommended both for internal and external use, and just start out using a little bit. (You'll want to be sure that she doesn't have an allergic reaction to it.)

Involve Her Breasts: When she is very aroused, you also might try adding some variety. *Variety* doesn't mean *fondle her breasts in a different way*, it means be inventive. For example, how about licking *under* her breasts, along the line where her breast joins her body. As you probably spend most of your time on the top side of her breasts, licking or lightly nipping the underside can be an exciting change. Similarly, try pinching her nipples between your thumb and forefinger, and then pull away from her body, thus pulling her breast(s) as you go. Not hard; not too much. You don't want to break the sensual mood you've developed. The message is that as arousal increases, your lady may ask for/want/

need stronger stimulation. Some of the books listed in Appendix A will provide examples of more adventurous forms of breast play.

Touching and Licking 101

Almost all of your touching and licking is designed to heighten the sexual mood of the evening and build towards her orgasm using stair-step techniques of build-up and fall-back cycles. To get the ball rolling, I suggest that you consider beginning your licking by hovering over her vulva for about five seconds before the first lick. Just stay there and breathe out — don't move at all. The hot, warm breath will feel great to her. For fun, you can even pant like a dog and sniff her. However, she's likely to erupt in laughter — which may be desirable, if you want to release her built-up tension.

Anyway, that first lick should be with a very relaxed tongue made as flat and as wide as you can make it. This is sometimes called the "St. Bernard" lick. She should be getting more and more excited with anticipation. After those five seconds elapse, make that lick very slow and very light, starting at the base of her vulva and ending on her mons.

Here's an important technique note: If you breathe *in,* while your face is near her vulva, then the air flowing over her may feel cold. To avoid this, move your head a little ways away from her to inhale the air in the room, then return to exhale hotly. Yes, I realize that you breathe an average of twelve times a minute. Rather than try to maintain that breathing pace, you might try taking much deeper breaths.

> **Tip #19:** There are going to be times during your evening's sexual play when you *do* want to break the pace you've established with your lady. While there are many, many ways to do that, one is to inhale the cooler room air while you are very close to her vulva, thus chilling the surface of her skin. At a minimum, she'll probably flinch; her reaction may be stronger than that. Again, you're breaking the mood — on purpose.

Get a Good Look: You might consider demonstrating your fondness for the area, particularly with a new sex partner, by isolating your playing field in order to make some appreciative comments. Comments such as: "What a lovely shape you have" will always be appreciated.

Starting to Lick: When you're just about ready to get down to serious licking, consider starting at her groin, the crease where her leg joins her body. By now, she should be dying for you to make your move. If you're doing it right, she'll be moaning and trying to force your head between her legs. Stretch this phase out until she looks as though she's been holding her breath for three days. (The worst thing that might happen is that she may begin to think that you've confused her groin for her vulva, but that will be worth a good laugh the next day.)

Before you lick, remember — the key word is *slow.* It's good to groan and moan, too. It shows you're enjoying it while it also sends nice vibrations right through her body.

> **Tip #20:** Try humming at strategic times to add sound vibration to your bag of tricks.

Your first few licks should be nice, sloppy St. Bernard licks before moving on. Take it really slowly — four seconds per lick. When making long bottom-to-top licks, please don't forget about the risks of fecal contamination and her vagina — stay well away from her anus.

This is a good time to figure out what kind of clit she has. If it's very sensitive, she'll probably convulse as you pass over it, and that means you're probably in for an easy ride. If there's no reaction when you graze over her clit, there is a chance that she's just not very sensitive there. But, there's an alternative: She could be very anxious about what you're starting to do, but because you didn't discuss this with her ahead of time, you have no way of knowing this. You have about 15 seconds to figure out if that's it, or if it's simply that she's not very verbal. Failure to quickly sort out the alternatives, can cause rapport problems for the rest of the evening.

To help you sort through the alternatives, you'll need to distinguish between "not very sensitive" and "not very verbal." Once you're focused on her clit, if she's not reacting pretty dramatically, you might want to ask her if there is something else you should be doing — or whether you should be doing this *differently.* As mentioned in the opening pages, women report that very few men seek feedback from them. If she's not reacting the way you would have thought she would, this is a good time to do some asking.

Intermission — Getting Feedback

And what *does* she think of your performance so far? Along your Path of Exploration, you will want to do some reality checking. Are you still the welcomed visitor or are you pushing your luck?

- Do you want me to go faster? Slower?
- Harder? Softer?
- Will you show me where to lick/touch?
- Would you prefer that I lick from top to bottom, from side to side, or in circles?
- Do you want long strokes or little flicks?
- How about here (i.e.: the crease between her body and her outer lips, or her outer/inner labia, or her perineum)?
- Do you want me to hold still for a minute? Tell me when to start again.
- Would you like me to try a little suction?
- Want me to keep going just like this…?

In addition to considering what she says, you must always be monitoring how she's responding.

- Nipples becoming darker and more erect?
- Pushing her pelvis in an encouraging way?
- Arching her back?
- Flexing her toes and fingers?
- Grabbing the sheets?
- Wanting to be in physical contact with you — holding your hand or forearm (if hand is not available)?

- Moaning and/or coaxing you on?
- Vaginal opening becoming dark and engorged with blood?
- Clitoris becoming more stiff and exposed?

Moving Right Along — Touching and Licking 201

While many women don't want you spending all your time on their clit, others **do** want you to spend a lot of time there. Again, ask for feedback from your lady. In general, though, I recommend that you spend most of your time doing other things: circle it, ride your tongue up and down between the inner and outer lips, suck it into your mouth. Pause after some licking to do some gentle pinching and pulling of the outer lips.

Try lightly tugging on her outer and/or inner lips: Speaking of pinching or pulling on her outer lips, let me begin by saying that some women really like this, and others don't like it. Still others start out not liking it, but really, really like it once they have been aroused. If done right, it can be very animalistic. Because she may get a thrill knowing that her sexuality is so primal that she's turned you into an animal, you may also want to try growling at this stage.

> **Tip #21:** You can quickly teach yourself to suck most of an outer lip (or the whole vulva), into your mouth. If you decide to try this, I then recommend that you bite down gently, but firmly enough so you've trapped the outer labial lip between your teeth. Pull away from her. Chances are, she'll either squeak or moan. If she squeaks, you're biting too hard. You don't necessarily have to stop; just release a little bit of your teeth grip. If she asks you to release most of the biting pressure, you can still get a good grip on her outer labial lip by sucking a bit harder.

Other options at this point include:

- Placing your lips around her clit, suck both her clit and some of the surrounding tissue into your mouth. You should easily develop the skill to push the clit back out and suck it back into your mouth in repeated cycles. Again, if she's an oral lady, this technique is bound to please her.

- Circle her vagina with your tongue, then ride your tongue up from the vaginal opening and stop when her clitoral bud is resting on the top of your tongue. You are now working in the area called the vestibule; the area above the vaginal opening and below the clit. Very small movements at that physical location should produce a lovely effect. Running your tongue up and down the vestibule should also produce a delightful experience for her.
- Combine sucking on her clit and flicking it with your tongue with placing two fingers over her vaginal opening and stroking gently. This should get her attention — but do not yet let your fingers enter her.
- In time with your carefully selected background music that has a strong beat, make your tongue very pointed and hard; lick from one side of her clitoral hood to the other, back and forth a few times. Intersperse this with very soft and gentle licking. Make your tongue very flat and soft. Start below her vaginal opening and end back up as far as you can go without landing on her mons. Yes, this was my recommendation for first starting out with your oral sex, but that certainly doesn't limit its use. The flat and soft tongue lick can be used at various times simply for the effect it produces.
- With two or three fingers inside her vagina, pretend your fingers are really an organic vibrator. Vibrate from side-to-side an up-and-down very quickly.
- While fingering her, consider licking, nibbling, or lightly biting her neck, tummy, or breasts.

Tip #22: Depending upon whether you are kneeling, lying on her left or right side, or lying between her legs when licking, you probably want to have fingers from one hand pulling one of her outer lips open. This way, you'll have more licking control. Use fingers from whichever hand is not occupied to touch lightly around her vaginal opening.

Tip #23: Continue doing the combo, above, until she has started to squirm sensually and/or moan piteously. Then, consider delivering a truly unexpected slap with the flat of your right hand onto her tummy or inner thigh — even on her entire vulva. Not too hard; you're going for a change of pace, here, you're not going for pain. With any luck at all, you should bring her right off the massage table or bed into a seated position.

At this point, your approved line is, "Oops, did I slap you too hard? Sorry. I guess we'll have to start over. I won't do it again." Be sure to look serious when you deliver these lines. She's likely to kill you if you smirk or laugh. Anyway, you then start your build-up all over again. After all, you're supposed to be *playing* with this lady, aren't you? As mentioned in the opening pages, the goal here is to get the woman to a certain level of stimulation, then back off a little, then rebuild to a slightly higher level of stimulation, then back off a little, then build up again. This can go on for quite a while, but at the end, once you've mastered this process, you just may be rewarded with one heck of a screaming orgasm.

Techniques to Fold into Your Licking Style

Tip #24: Clits come in a wide variety of shapes, sizes, and sensitivities, but that doesn't really tell you much. All of them want to be treated slowly and gently at the beginning, but the only way to tell if you can go fast at the end is by reading her reactions. Please keep in mind that flinching means "take it easy" and "*ohmygodohmygodohmygod*" means "keep doing it." Also, some women are more tactile than verbal, so if she's pulling your head tightly between her legs, you're also on the right track, whether or not she's moaning.

Clits that need a serious going over: Some women like their clits played with fairly rigorously. These situations are often a great deal of fun because you can be creative. For example, you can pretend that your tongue is the bad cop and the clit is the babe who killed your partner. First, separate her from her buddies (the lips) and suck her right up into your mouth. Now she's on your turf. Keep her erect by creating an air-tight vacuum chamber in your mouth. Now, slap her with one big tongue boink. After a few teasers and swirling circles, rat-a-tat-tat her senseless like a boxer whacking a speed bag. If her reactions tell you that this is too much, ease up on the interrogation and go back to the St. Bernard licks (wide, flat tongue). The vacuum is a great way to bring her to orgasm, but it's a bit much sometimes, so mix things up with some circles around the clit and some penetrating tongue action.

As her arousal increases, go back to the vacuum and tongue smacking interspersed with some up-and-down licking all over the area; this is another time to throw in some St. Bernard licks and some side-to-side licks. Be careful, here; you won't want to do anything wild. Just make some gentle movement, only an inch or so each way. Sometimes, if she is just on the edge of an orgasm, you may feel her starting to shake. This is good. Be repetitive. Do not be creative right now. You've almost brought her home; this is not the time to change tactics.

- ***Extra tip:*** To keep the rhythm going, synchronize your licking to the music you're playing. If you don't like playing music during sex, try repeating a chant in your head that goes with the movement of your tongue (hi-yi-yi-ya, hi-yi-yi-ya, hi-yi-yi-ya). Any inconsistent action may cause her to come back into her head to figure out what isn't quite right. If that happens, it is likely to stop her progression to orgasm — or at least set you back a few minutes, which, at this stage, can be bad for morale. (By way of more formal wording, changing your actions, being out of sync with the music, or a dramatic change in the beat of your licking, may cause what is termed a "state change" (mentioned in the definitions section of Chapter One). That is, you're changing her state-of-being from a *feeling* state to a *thinking* state. If some of her non-verbal signals change suddenly, you've got a good clue about what just happened.)

- ***Important:*** Keep going a few seconds after her orgasm — but don't hit her clit. Now, you should circle around her clitoral area and slowly bring her down. If you keep going, you're likely to feel her hands come down from above and lay you off. That may well be a sign that you're not paying enough attention to her reactions. Remember, at this point, all her erogenous zones are hypersensitive. Also remember, she's basking in the glow of an orgasm and probably wants to revel in the feelings without having to think about what you're now doing to her. Again, if she puts her hand on your head in this manner, she's had to come back into her head (thinking state).

- ***Important additional tip:*** If your lady is multi-orgasmic, she may or may not want to go directly for a second orgasm. If you think that she does want you to start up again, you'll still want to give her a brief quiet period. As I repeatedly stress, women vary widely in their preferences, so it's up to you to figure out what she wants. If you're not sure what to do, slow down for a minute or two and start back up again until the magic hands come down to push you away.

Clits that don't like heavy duty action: Some ladies don't like their clits to be singled out and battered around. She may be new to intense oral play, or she may simply not like it. Although infrequent, on some ladies, you're likely to find that their clits are not particularly sensitive, so you're not advancing your cause by lingering overlong on it. If you run into this situation, just do casual St. Bernard licks combined with some of the previously discussed fingering techniques until she orgasms, pure and simple.

Now, if you've been licking/fingering/vibrating her for a long period and she doesn't come to a climax, you may think that you're failing her. That's probably not her thought. First, some women take a very long time to relax enough to get really turned on; second, she may be non-orgasmic (libido lowered because of medications, still a bit anxious about being with you, psychological stress as a result of not having orgasms with a man, etc); third, there's a chance that you're one of the first guys she's been with that will go so long with this kind of oral sex play and she's just loving it (in which case, sticking it out just may lead to delicious payback when/if the roles are reversed).

Finis: At some point, she'll let you know that she's now satisfied and that you are to stop because she wants to take a break. This can be communicated either orally (she'll tell you to stop) or physically (her whole body relaxes and she becomes non-responsive to your advances). At this stage, she's going to want you out of there. Among other reasons, the whole area is now hypersensitive and your touching/licking is not pleasurable any more. A somewhat risky alternative to leaving her alone at this point is to see how she likes it if you stick out your relaxed tongue and very gently lay it down on her closed outer lips. Make sure you don't move it, as that can actually annoy her. Just let it sit there for about thirty seconds.

Few evenings end at this point. If she is still aroused and active after orgasm, and if intercourse was planned, skip the activities described in the preceding paragraph and start that part of your sexual play.

Bonus Tips

Getting Fired

In some of the paragraphs, above, I've mentioned her hands coming down and gently pushing you away after an orgasm. "Getting fired" is very different. If two hands suddenly drop from the sky and start pulling you up when you're in the middle of your cunnilingus play, you've just been sacked. She may tell you she never climaxes from that, anyway, but the truth is more likely to be that for this particular lady, you're just not doing it correctly. Either ask her to instruct you, or just go back to fingering (or intercourse) and look at the whole thing as a learning experience. If she's willing to guide you, then let her know that comments such as, "Slow down you're going too fast…" or "Yeah-right-there-like-that…" or "Oh-that's-perrrrrfect" can be very helpful.

The Seven Worst Cunnilingus Mistakes

Making like a gynecologist: Sure, you're curious about what a new partner's private parts look like up close; go ahead and take a good look. But don't spread her labia open so wide that she feels as though she's getting her annual pelvic exam. There's nothing romantic about a gynecological exam. Just use your fingertips to gently hold back her outer lips, take your look — and then lightly slip your tongue in there. (I know; previously I suggested that you start with the St. Bernard lick. You're in charge of how you start out; I can only suggest some alternatives.)

Blowing air into her vagina: This is a problem; this is risky. Blowing air into her vagina actually involves health risks. This is important enough to stress it in a safety warning.

> **Safety Warning #10:** Do not form a seal around your partner's vagina with your lips and blow into it. Blowing lightly or breathing on and around her vulva is hot, but blowing air **into** her vagina with your mouth (or with an aerosol can such as whipped cream) is dangerous. Safety-guru Jay Wiseman comments: "The air can get into her venous blood system and travel to her lungs, causing an air-bubble-induced pulmonary embolism, which can be a Very Bad Thing."

Women are most at risk when their pelvic vessels are enlarged (meaning, increased blood supply to the vagina) due to arousal, some forms of trauma, or pregnancy. In some cases, the woman (and her fetus) may experience complications of various sorts resulting from this act. As Jay mentioned in the safety warning, in extraordinary cases, some of these women (and her fetus, if she's pregnant) could die if the embolism were to travel to her lungs.

Lapping like a dog: It's good to lick, and it's good to keep your tongue loose and relaxed. But don't get sloppy or slobbery. Use a little restraint, and (unless you know your lady really likes it) don't start to act like a panting dog. If your oral technique reminds her of her pet Collie, that's unlikely to be a turn-on. At worst, she may either start giggling and break her relaxed, sensual mood, or she may suddenly come present (also breaking her relaxed sensual mood) and say forcefully, "Stop that!" (Recall the discussion of "state change.")

Clit hickeys: If you simply *must* leave your mark, do it on her arm, breast (where it won't show) or thigh. Don't clamp your mouth around her clit and suck it like a vacuum cleaner. Strong suction on her clit isn't going to feel very good to her, and it's likely to hurt.

Cunnilingus after drinking heavily: Heavy drinking and cunnilingus *do not* mix. To do a good job down there, you need to be able to pay attention and coordinate your tongue action with vibrators or with finger action. If you've been drinking heavily, you might pass out, and that pretty much guarantees you won't get another date with her. It is your job to maintain a sexual play setting that is safe, responsible, and consensual. Trying to do the kind of sexual playing described in this book after an evening of heavy drinking, or after recreational drug use, is none of these things.

Jabbing and stabbing: If you're insistently jabbing and poking your pointy tongue onto her clit or into her vagina, chances are that she views this just as creepy and uncomfortable as she would if you were sticking your tongue in her ear or behaving this way in French kissing. It makes you come off as overeager and unskilled. Relax your tongue and take your time. Gently caress her clit and let her bring her privates to you.

Tongue exhaustion: Tongue exhaustion is the number-one cause of abandoning cunnilingus — but, there are some ways to avoid this problem.

- You can use your tongue as an inanimate object. Stick it out as far as it can go and tense it. Then move it around the inner workings of her vulva using your neck muscles. Remember, use small motions; don't try big motions with this move.
- You can use your fingers and toys while you give your mouth a rest.
- Using the beat of music that is playing to time your actions; when the music changes to another tune, use the few seconds between CD music cuts to stop that action completely. When the new tune starts to play (with a new beat, in most cases), change what you were doing to something slightly different. Give your tongue a break.

Remember also, that some gentle pinching, poking, pulling, and slapping needs to be worked in with all the licking and fingering. Think *sensation play,* and provide her with new sensations. This is *critical* to help your partner avoid desensitization from all the licking and sucking. Again, you should have already cleared these types of play techniques with her in pre-session negotiations.

By way of conclusion, cunnilingus is an art form. As with all art forms, it requires substantial practice and involves asking partners what you're doing right and wrong. Fortunately, practice of this kind can be terrifically fun.

Health Considerations and Oral Sex

Ahem. Oral sex is not a risk-free adventure.

Here is an open letter posted on the Internet that is very relevant at this point in the book. It is by Charles Moser, Ph.D., M.D., a specialist in sexually transmitted infections.

Dear folks,

I want to make a few comments about STIs and STI testing discussion.

First, we are no longer calling it STD (Sexually Transmitted Diseases), but STI (Sexually Transmitted Infections). Under this new view, many new things are STIs, including a cold and or flu. This means that when someone says they have been checked out and are "clean," it is a meaningless statement unless you know what orifices have been checked for what bugs. Not to mention when they were checked and when was their last possible exposure.

For obvious reasons we cannot do a scientific experiment to expose a group of people to an STI, and then see how long it takes for the test to turn positive. So all the arguments about when the test turns positive are somewhat arbitrary best guesses. There are also differences among people; two people infected at the same time — even by the same person — may become symptomatic or test positive at different times. Although it may be possible to detect an HIV infection in 10 days, not everyone infected will be positive in 10 days. The experts have designated 6 months as the arbitrary limit, but more than 95% (if memory serves me) become positive by 6 weeks.

In medicine, we never say never. It is true that oral sex is a very poor way to transmit HIV, but it probably has happened. Hepatitis C is rarely sexually transmitted, but sharing bloody toys can increase the infection risk significantly. Herbert: it appears that this textbox line cannot be removed in Word. Please eremove it, as there is no break between these parts.

> The analogy that I like to use is that of driving a car. If you do not want to die in a car wreck, do not get in a car. If you like the convenience of tooling around town, there are many things you can do to reduce your risk. Do not drink and drive, wear your seat belts, keep your car in good repair, obey traffic laws, etc. All these things reduce your risk, but not to zero. You have to be comfortable with the level of risk. You are much more likely to die in a car crash than get HIV via oral sex or Hep C by vaginal or anal sex, but the risk is not zero. Unfortunately, no one can quantify the risk accurately.
>
> Doing safer sex is a good idea, but condoms break and condoms do not protect completely against some diseases (Herpes). If you like sex, enjoy, but like everything else there is always some danger. No one can guarantee complete safety, but we do not seem to worry about getting hit by lightning, maybe a similar attitude is helpful with STIs. Hope this helps. I can answer specific questions if anyone has them.
>
> Take care,
>
> Charles Moser, Ph.D., M.D.

For more details about specific STI risks and sexual practices, please go to the CDC's website (Center for Disease Control and Prevention — http://www.cdc.gov).

Special Note on Brushing Your Teeth Before Sex

Don't do it. You'll make a zillion little cuts in your mouth and vastly increase disease transmission risk. (See: http://www.aidsmap.com then go to "oral sex" and do a search on "teeth".)

Chapter Summary

This is the first of the real *techniques* chapters in this book. I opened by noting that your skills in this area will stand you apart from other men. In my experience, women remember and seek out men who can demonstrate their experience with cunnilingus.

Next, I provided a section containing some material that you should know before starting down this path. This included not only your psychological state, but also *her* psychological state. I spent quite a bit of time, there, as I felt that readers would benefit from reading some comments from ladies who had strong feelings about this subject. From there, I discussed the delicate issues of a lady's odor and taste, then covered the importance of discussing (negotiating) some of the details of your intended sexual activity before beginning your evening. I mentioned that *nobody likes surprises,* and that some of this play — if not pre-negotiated — is likely to surprise the lady and cause her to rethink the relationship.

I reviewed not only the importance of knowing how to kiss, but also the importance of making sure your lady is always well-lubricated. Next was a quick review about learning where to touch your lady, then some thoughts about your respective physical positions during sexual play.

From there, a substantial portion of this chapter was devoted to an in-depth discussion of techniques of oral sexual play — how to start licking and how to progress to advanced licking. Next, I stressed the critical importance of getting feedback from your lady. This is a theme that is woven into almost every aspect of this book, for it can't be overstated.

The last pages of this chapter reviewed more advanced techniques for oral sexual play, and gave you some extra information that may help you avoid common problems that could arise during cunnilingus.

Chapter Ten

Anal Play and Related Topics

Safety Warning #6, Repeated a Third Time, with Slight Modification: If you're playing anally with multiple partners with whom you are not fluid bonded, and if you're using sex toys that have a porous surface (such as plastic, rubber, or silicone toys), you ***must*** cover them with a condom. You must do this to avoid the possibility of contaminating them with body fluids that could contain STIs. Many sex toys can retain body fluids unless you're disinfecting them with some kind of medical cleanser — previously discussed.

Analingus involves a variety of techniques to stimulate your lady's anal area. This includes kissing, licking, fingering, and sliding the tongue in and out of the anus. Rectal fingering is not, strictly speaking, part of analingus. Pleasure from being rimmed comes from the sensitive nerve endings surrounding the anus that are typically stimulated by the tongue and lips. The pleasure can be so intense that it can sometimes be the only sexual stimulation she needs to reach orgasm. In a general sense, you're likely to find that women either love this or won't even consider it.

Note: Even if this book was covering penile penetration, I would not cover anal intercourse. There are great books out there that do an outstanding job.

On Cleanliness and Fetishes – A Short Detour

In this country, bathing is so common that one seldom thinks about it. This book assumes that you and your lady have had showers fairly recently. But some people may not want their partner to bathe.

While *not bathing* for a number of days may sound outrageous to most readers, please recall that Napoleon Bonaparte, as he was about to return from the Russian front, famously wrote to his wife, Josephine, saying, "I'm coming home, don't bathe." Some percentage of any population will have some kind of fetish you've never heard of — and for many of you, you'd just as soon leave it that way. But what about the lady you're going to be playing with? What might be *her* fetishes?

Now, while not related to this section on *cleanliness,* I've listed examples of some of the more tame sexual fetishes out there. An Internet search for *sexual fetishes* can give you many, many others.

- Sexual arousal is connected with their partner being dressed in gorgeous latex clothing.
- Sexual arousal must start with the woman's bottom, not her front.
- Sexual arousal consists of admiring, stroking, and licking a woman's high heels.
- Sexual arousal to orgasm comes from being spanked in a role play situation.
- A sexual evening almost *requires* a formal dinner service where he's in a tux (or equivalent) and his partner is dressed in a corset or cincher and bra, garter belt, hose, and high heels. But no panties.

Remember, it takes all kinds to make a horse race. Message: Be respectful of others' fetishes — and consider exploring your own. If you can think of it, chances are that there's a group out there that's actually doing it.

Details of Play

Anal Finger Play

If you are dealing with a particularly saucy vixen, she may want some anal touching or even penetration. If you're just doing a little bit of anal exploration, you can probably get by with a *finger cot* for your thumb (available from drug stores). However, if you are actually considering entering her rectum, or if you intend to wander from her anus to her vulva, I strongly recommend that you put on **two** latex gloves, one over the other. This way, when you wish to change back from anal fingering to vaginal fingering, you can simply slip off the outer glove and still remain gloved in case you want to return to anal play in a few minutes. (I discuss the need for gloves for vaginal fingering in the next chapter.)

If you're new to this, I recommend you start out with a finger cot on your thumb. This is probably the most comfortable initial approach. Please keep in mind that anal play (particularly if she is new to this) may split her sensory attention and thus should most often be saved until you're near the end of your licking and vibrator play. A split in her sensory attention causes a state change. When you start playing around her anus, she will immediately move from a *feeling* to a *thinking* state. If she's new to this, you're likely tripping over all kinds of cultural taboos, and she's going to have to work through them before she can relax.

Incidentally, if you're trying to introduce anal play as part of your routine play, try introducing it just before orgasm, it should substantially increase the intensity of her orgasm and accompanying scream. As an added benefit, you should be able to induce a Pavlovian response (an *anchor* in the language of NLP and hypnosis) that could last for the rest of the relationship. That is, she may come to associate anal sex with extreme pleasure. Once again, you must use a finger cot or rubber glove for these kinds of activities, or risk getting fecal matter in her vagina if you return to vaginal play. As stated previously, this is a serious no-no. You must be very, very careful not to touch the vaginal area after touching the anal area. Cots and rubber gloves make this separation much easier.

As I've said frequently, this book does not cover intercourse, either anal or vaginal. There are very competent books out there that discuss vaginal and anal intercourse in excellent detail. This chapter contains only discussions of fingering techniques. It starts out purely about anal fingering but ends up combining anal and vaginal fingering.

The best position for this group of techniques would have the woman on her knees with the man kneeling behind her.

- Keeping my health commentaries in mind, consider circling around her anus with one double-gloved hand while playing with her vagina with your other hand. Note: This is much easier to accomplish if your lady is on her knees.

- Once she's accommodated to this, you might want to enter her rectum a bit. As I keep saying, you really *must* use a finger cot or a latex glove. In each of those cases, remember to use a water-based or vegetable-based lube for anal play.

Given the nature of your lady, she should either be fabulously turned on or asking you to stop. If she's Fabulously Turned On, you can segue into our next section. If she's Fabulously Turned Off, you get to start all over. Sigh.

> **Tip #25:** Double-glove one hand so that after some anal play you can strip off the glove and, still gloved, then return to her vulva. If you're experienced at vaginal fisting, this might be a good time to start thinking about that.

You may find that your sexual play partner(s) enjoy it when you insert your gloved thumb inside her rectum while two or three fingers are inside her vagina. Again, this activity is easier to accomplish if your lady is kneeling. Your fingers will almost touch, being separated by the top lining of her rectum and the bottom lining of her vagina. You might consider pulling your thumb in and out, *slowly,* taking care not to contaminate her vaginal area with any body fluids on your thumb.

Now, this group of techniques is a bit more advanced than the previous group, and delves more deeply into techniques that combine anal and vaginal fingering. Your lady should probably remain on her knees, but as you become adept at these techniques, you may prefer her to be on her tummy. You **must** be gloved for this, and — preferably — double-gloved.

- Your thumb is in her rectum, but your fingers are only on the edge of her vagina. Move in and out with your thumb. Very, very gently run a finger or two around her vaginal opening. In many women, this is easier to accept than when your fingers are actually moving around inside her vagina, so this is a good starting point.

- Your thumb is in her rectum and your fingers are pointing downward with your index finger resting in her slit. Tense your arm (make a muscle) and vibrate up-and-down very rapidly. You may only be moving your hand up-and-down ½ inch or less; this is not a large-movement technique. In the alternative, relax your arm and use a pendulum motion with your index finger, back and forth across her clitoral hood while your thumb is making circles inside her rectum.
- Once she's comfortable with this action, you can probably get some pretty vigorous vaginal play going. You have a choice, at this point. You can move your fingers that are inside her vagina and your thumb that is inside her rectum at the same speed, or you can establish one speed for your thumb and another much faster speed for her vaginal stimulation. This is the old "patting your head while rubbing your tummy" test. (If you're going to try this fingering with different speeds, then consider something like five vaginal movements to every one entry or exit stroke of your thumb.) Yes, I know; this takes some practice.

Butt Plugs

As their use is pretty obvious, I'll do no more than give you photos of three sizes of rubber butt plugs and one glass plug. While certainly not for everyone, many ladies are particularly partial to these sex toys.

Bringing it All Together — The Triple Whammy

First, get into this position:

- Your lady is on her back.
- You are lying on your tummy slightly astride her at about a 45-degree angle (your buttocks about even with her head, and your head is between her legs).
- You can be lying on whichever side of her feels best for you.
- While your head is between her legs, both of your hands are free for Other Things.

From this position, consider simultaneously fingering her anus (with the gloved hand) and her vagina (with your other hand), all this while licking her clit and the surrounding tissues.

I think you'll be delighted with the way this gets her erotic attention. Think of it as *Sexual Pleasing-401.*

Health Issues

Fingering Issue

Once again, when using your fingers, be careful not to stroke directly from the anus to the vagina. If you are directly stimulating the anal area, you must take care to keep those fingers separate from fingers playing in her vaginal area.

Licking (rimming) Issues

Rimming — tonguing your partner's anus — is certainly adored by many and abhorred by many. It is an unsafe activity unless you use a barrier. There are many health problems that can result from practicing unsafe rimming, because of the presence of bacteria, viruses, or parasites on the anus or in the rectum. These include Hepatitis A and C, HPV, intestinal parasites, and other sexually transmitted infections. Applying your mouth to her genitals immediately after licking her anus can inadvertently introduce the bacterium *Escherichia coli* (often referred to as *E. coli*) into the urethra, causing a urinary tract infection. If introduced into the vagina, it can cause a vaginal infection. HIV/AIDS is not believed to be easily transmitted through rimming, but experts assert that there is a theoretical risk of acquiring HIV from rimming. CAN YOU FIX THE JUSTIFICATION HERE? (http://www.dph.sf.ca.us/sfcityclinic/drk/hivaids7.asp)

Frequent rimming with casual partners increases the health risks associated with the practice. Generally, people carrying infections that may be passed on during rimming will appear healthy. By the way, parasites may be found in someone's feces if they ate badly cooked meat. Remember, STI testing is irrelevant when thinking about problems with amoebas, parasites, shigella, salmonella, or E. coli. STI tests aren't intended to identify any of these.

Hepatitis A may appear in feces if the infected person has eaten contaminated food — the source of which is usually associated with unclean health practices of restaurant staff. It is rare to catch Hepatitis C from your partner through rimming, although it is possible if the rimmee has trace amounts of infected blood in his/her anus or in feces. As various kinds of bugs make their home in the gastro-intestinal tract, you must also be aware that your licking can expose you to intestinal infections. For example, there is some risk of exposure to parasitic protozoa such as a*moebas* (sometimes picked up from unwashed vegetables — generally outside the US) or *Giardia lamblia* (most prevalent in this country in high-mountain streams where the water that is feeding the streams has traversed elk or deer fields that are littered with fecal matter). On the bacterial front, you could be exposed either to *shigella,* to *salmonella,* or to *campylobacter.* While not typically residing in the anus or rectum, these infections can be living in the upper digestive tract — especially the bacteria or the cysts of the protozoa — and are eliminated from the body via the fecal route. Thus, unprotected rimming can present a health risk for you.

And that can be a problem. According to Jack Morin, author of Anal Pleasure and Health (1984), studies in the gay communities of New York, Los Angeles, and San Francisco show that between 40-80% of sexually active gay men may have amoebas or giardia parasites. He goes on to point out that this makes them far-and-away the most common of the intestinal infections among men in the US. Worse, about half the time, someone who has caught these bugs may experience rather tame symptoms — such as fever, cramping, or diarrhea — rather than more traditional signs of infection. Thus, someone may be infected and not know it.

While this may be too much information, medical detection of the presence of amoebas or giardia require repeated tests. Single-stool samples examined by pathologists will only reveal these diseases 45-60% of the time. Morin reports that to get 90% accuracy, you have to donate three samples, tested a few days apart.

The association of rimming and unprotected anal intercourse with AIDS is well-known, so I won't go over it, here. An Internet search provides many authoritative citations.

Some safer sex options include:

- A dental dam
- Non-microwaveable plastic wrap

- Seriously limiting the number of partners with whom you are rimming

Chapter Summary

After a short detour delving into fetishes, I described some techniques for anal fingering that also included some concurrent vaginal fingering. I then closed with a critical discussion of health issues, as this activity, more than any other type of sexual activity discussed in this book, carries the greatest health risk. A section on safer sex options then followed.

I concluded with a short paragraph about combining everything you've learned in this book.

Chapter Eleven

Fingering Techniques

> "The first thing you need to do is look at your hands in a new way — not for throwing a football, not for using power tools (well, we take that back), not for flipping channels, but as versatile tools of love. Most guys use their fingers like they use their penis. Don't be silly. You castrate the power of your hands when you do that!" Lesbian Sex Secrets for Men, p. 122.

I cannot agree with this more strongly. Men have so much more sensitivity and control with their fingers than they do with their penis, that there is simply no comparison. While I certainly don't want to take anything away from sexual intercourse, my own experience is that you can get more reactions from your lady using your fingers and tongue than your penis. And — hear this — once you start putting your pre-intercourse emphasis on licking, fingering, and vibrators, you're going to find that your ladies (when asked) will tell you that you're one of fewer than 2% of all their lifetime sexual play partners who can play sexually with them this way. And they'll often ask to come back — which is a treat.

> **Safety Warning #11:** If you're going inside your lady's vagina, wear gloves. If you insist on going in without gloves, then I strongly urge you to trim, buff, and scrub your fingernails before you start. Not to be too extreme about this, you might consider scrubbing fingernails with 90% alcohol (90% because that's about the strongest alcohol on the market) or other hand sanitizer, and then rinsing them off. You'll become a believer the first time you face the doctor and medication bills from having given your lady bacterial vaginosis. Unfortunately, this is the voice of experience talking, not some theoretical concept or urban legend.

Rules for Early-Stage Fingering

I know, you don't like rules. Or, you have your own rules. Remember, though, you're trying to develop a set of skills that evoke specific responses from your lady; that's hard to do if your sexual play is somewhat random, or created on-the-spot with each new partner.

Rule One: Let Her Instruct You About Her Body

When you start out with a new lady, you will win points if you ask her to take your finger and place it where she receives the most enjoyment. It may take you some time to learn how to relinquish control over your hand and let the lady guide you — it's not as easy as it sounds, if you're a dominant male. Here, you should be alert: Is she barely touching the area or pushing down with hard movements? Is she going up-and-down, or using some other pattern, such as sideways or diagonally? Is she focused on a particular area of her vulva, or does she wander all about? Ask her, specifically, how she likes her clit played with. If you are comfortable together, you also might ask her to show you how she masturbates.

This is exactly the time to determine where, in the area called the *vestibule,* she likes to be touched. (Remember, the vestibule is the area of very soft, smooth skin that starts above her vaginal opening and ends just under her clitoral bud.) Some women are more sensitive in the area above the vaginal opening up to their urethra; some women prefer that you stroke the area above the urethra up to the clit (the U-spot). Some women don't particularly differentiate between the two areas.

> **Tip #26:** Some women are more sensitive on one side of their anatomy than on another side. This applies to the clit and clitoral hood, as well as their inner lips. This is why it's so important when starting with a new partner to let her show you what pleases her.

Rule Two: Start Out Slowly

At this point, keep away from her vagina. Consider starting out by lying between her legs and placing the palm of your hand over her entire vulva and either vibrating your hand or gently twisting it. Check with her to determine her preferred motion. You might try catching her clitoral shaft between your first and second fingers and simply rotating your hand from side-to-side a little bit at about one turn per second (yes, that slowly). You may also wish to hold your fingers still and only rotate your palm slightly — while lightly clamping her clitoral shaft. This last movement is best performed if your lady is on her back and you are lying between her legs with your fingers (catching her hood) pointed upward. This is a good general warm-up. Next, run your fingers over her outer lips and slit — teasing her before you start putting fingers in there.

Rule Three: Don't Touch a Dry Clit or a Dry Vagina

We've been over this one. Use some lube (or saliva). You may wish to try some sugar-free lube. Be attentive always to keep vulva-related objects well lubricated: clit, vestibule, and vagina. If you need a memory-jogger, think: *well-oiled machine.* For the vast majority of women, having a dry finger inside their vaginas won't make them wet, it will only irritate them and start them thinking that they must have been out of their mind to agree to have sex with you.

Rule Four: Relax Your Fingers and Don't Move Them Too Much

You're going to need to learn ways of relaxing your hand/fingers; you're going to need to practice making very, very small movements, whether it's playing with her clit and clitoral hood, entering her vaginal canal, or stroking her spongy tissue. This is a time for exploration. More importantly, this is the time when you're moving more slowly than she really wants.

That's okay, because this way she'll be thinking that she wants you to do *more* rather than less. Remember: Teasing = good; going too fast = bad.

Rule Five: Don't Go Straight for Her Clit

I've said this before, and I mean it: This is a pleasuring and teasing game, not a conquest game. You should be trailing your fingers down her stomach, up her leg, and inner thighs. You should caress an outer labial lip, then skip across her slit and caress the other side. Repeat. Repeat. Repeat. And keep away from focusing on her nipples; you just may discover that nipple stroking is more a *guy thing* than a *girl thing*. Sure, the nipples are sensitive; but, as is often said, too much of a good thing is still too much. The skin of her breasts (particularly their undersides) and stomach could use some much-wanted attention, too. Anyway, you've probably run across many women who would prefer that you keep away from their nipples, at least for starters.

By the way, your prior ladies may not have tried to limit your breast fondling, even if they didn't particularly enjoy all the time you spent doing it. This is not only because our culture is focused on female breasts (so men and women expect lots of breast play before sex), but also because the lady is also interested in showing you a good time and she assumes that all the breast play pleases you. Once again, this is an area you might wish to discuss with your lady/ladies.

Rule Six: Ask for Feedback

I know; I keep beating you over the head with this one. But, it's the key to success with this book, and especially with fingering techniques. Because women have fewer nerve endings in their vaginas than in most of the surrounding tissue, many women can't *exactly* tell what you're doing in there. Much of your feeling around inside her vagina is translated by her as *pressure.* This reemphasizes the need to check in often: "Right now, my fingers are pointed down, do you like it?" or "I'm moving my fingers across your cervix; what do you think? Too deep? Deeper? This fast? How about if I lick a little as we start out with fingering?" (She's likely to be surprised that you've asked her; you've just set yourself apart from virtually all of her prior sexual partners.) Anyway, getting back to our theme, you'll need to adjust your *technique* with each of your sex partners. As I keep stressing, women drive differently. It's your task to figure out how to drive her before you crash and burn.

Rule Seven: Don't Rub Her as Hard as You Rub Yourself

Men — far more than women — tend to be much more vigorous and forceful during masturbation. In early-stage sexual play, you're likely to get much more mileage by circling her clit with your tongue or fingers than you'll get by starting out directly on her clit. You are likely to get even more points out of almost touching her clit — by brushing by it vvveeerrrryyyy lightly and then moving on (back to body stroking). You're likely to find this method to be superior to direct clitoral stimulation in early-stage activities. You may want to go on like this for five to ten minutes. After all, you've got a whole Woman in front of you who will let you touch her everywhere. Why hurry?

Rule Eight: Women Vary in How They Like You to Start Out

In your pre-negotiation discussions, you'll gain points by asking your lady how she likes to start out her sexual evenings. Does she like to know in advance, or does she prefer spontaneity? Does she want to participate in planning the sex scene, or does pre-planning ruin it for her? And, what about the intensity you use to start out? Some like you to be forceful and to "take" them. Others will want you to be gentle and to worship them. Many won't have thought this through very thoroughly and will have trouble answering a direct question on the subject. In this case, consider her indecision to be an opportunity to demonstrate your range of starting moves, while asking for feedback — which should be a lot of good fun, yes?

The only caution at this stage is to recall the admonition back in Rule One: Don't start by sticking your finger in her vagina. The author of Lesbian Sex Secrets for Men notes that this demonstrates over eagerness. This form of over eagerness is the most common practice among men, but is one of the *least appreciated* actions among women.

> **Tip #27:** "Taking" the woman or "worshiping" the woman are all common role play activities in the world of adventurous sex. If you think you'd enjoy some role play, please pick up a copy of Patrick Califia's excellent book Sensuous Magic: a Guide to S/M for Adventurous Couples, 2001.

Rule Nine: Play Doctor

This is an excellent time to leisurely explore the feel of her vaginal walls. Spongy tissue on top? How much? Is spongy tissue also felt when you insert your fingers pointing downward (perineal sponge)? Where is her cervix? (This can vary somewhat among women.) By the way, the authors of Lesbian Sex Secrets for Men urge men at this stage to start whispering sweet nothings into their lady's ear — including what you're feeling as you're starting to probe around in there. They point out that because of the often-limited number of nerve endings inside the vagina, she'll start to learn her body better if you can say what you're doing and ask for feedback.

Rule Ten: Enter Her Vagina Slowly

I should add, slowly and *gently.* Consider starting by entering a partner's vagina less than an inch and wiggling one or two fingers a very little amount. Then move up with one finger to massage her spongy tissue.

Rule Eleven: Have Her Go to the Bathroom

Because some of the techniques described below involve applying substantial pressure to your lady's spongy tissue, and as the spongy tissue surrounds her urethra, it will be normal for her to want to stop your actions in order to go to the bathroom. If she urinates before you begin your evening, she is more likely to get through your intense fingering without discomfort.

We'll stop with Rules, at this point.

Fingering Techniques

Basic Fingering

This is far from an exhaustive list; it's just some ideas you may not have considered. Also, this should start you thinking of some more possible combinations and permutations of your own design. If you have some favorites that you would like me to include in future editions of this book, my email appears at the end of the final chapter. I'll be sure to cite you, if you wish.

The bulleted points that follow presume that the woman is on her back.

- From any position that will allow you to do so, trap her clitoral shaft between your well-lubricated first and second fingers and flick those fingers up and down, much as you would kick your feet if you were swimming.
- From this same position, capture her shaft and clit between those fingers and pull gently away from her body.
- Similar position, but this time place your middle finger on her clit and capture her outer lips between your first and third fingers and pull gently (or not-so-gently once she's aroused) away from her body.
- Now, take a position so that you're lying or kneeling beside her, facing her head. If you're right-handed, you would probably be on her right side. Move your hand so that all your fingers (held together, pointed straight out) are able to enter her slit. Now wiggle your fingers, thus stimulating her shaft, clit, vestibule, and vaginal opening all at one time.
- With your lady still on her back, change your position so that you are lying next to her, but at about a 45-degree angle with your head between her open legs. Both of your hands have access to her vulva. Run the index finger of one hand gently up and down her well-lubricated clitoral hood, stopping every-so-often to graze her clitoral bud. Use your left hand to do some vaginal fingering while stimulating other parts of her vulva with your tongue.

- Next, use your index and third fingers of one hand to spread her outer lips wide open. Use the other hand to run a well-lubricated finger up and down her vestibule and up and down either side of her clitoral shaft. Don't always hit her clit on the upward stroke. Sometimes you should jump over her clit and land on her clitoral shaft. Again, teasing is a good thing. Sometimes you should lift your finger and allow it to hover for a while, and then tap down on her clit a few times. At this point, you might try saying something like, "Hmmm, it's time to see how you're coming." You then may want to shift your body position slightly so your head is between her legs. Now, exhale hot breath on the widely exposed sensitive skin. This is a "haaaaaaa" exhalation, not a blowing action. You may only have two seconds of breath in you. (Please remember to turn your head away when you suck the air back into your lungs; failure to do so will immediately chill the area you just warmed up.)

> **Tip #28:** As with virtually all aspects of sex play, try not to be too predictable. If you're too predictable, you risk taking the excitement and adventure out of the evening, and this is not good.

- Still with two hands active, start using circular motions around and very slightly inside her vaginal opening while stroking her clitoral shaft.

- Find the position that suits you, and then stroke her perineum while also playing at the entrance to her vagina. (Remember your health-safety issues when playing near the anus.)

Advanced Fingering

This group of suggestions simply won't work if you're just starting your evening of sex. In chess-speak, these are all "early end-game" techniques that are meant to transition to special techniques for producing orgasm or female ejaculation. You'll have to wait a few pages for those.

You'll recall that I mentioned that once aroused, ladies usually want (or at least can tolerate) more forceful stimulation. These techniques are designed for that stage of your sexual evening. Some of these advanced techniques involve anchoring her heightened sexual mood in order to be able to help her to access these erotic sensations at other times.

Lady on her back:

- While your lady is on her back, intersperse some fairly light slapping to her inner thighs or to her vulva, itself. Using feedback, you'll be able to tell how hard to slap her. Used sparingly, this is a good state-change technique to slow down action when she is very near her climax. You might consider one, single, medium slap interspersed a few times with other techniques in this group.

- You're likely to get serious sighs and thrashing from this one; and this one won't appeal to everyone. But, I will say — you can become known for this move. I've put it in the "advanced" section, but it can be used either as an opening move or as a way to get a huge boost in her arousal level. If you've been licking and fingering away and you hit one of the times that you've backed her off, wiggle down below her feet (or turn your body 180-degrees) and without warning, put her big toe in your mouth. For nearly all women, this will produce an *instant positive reaction.* And I mean positive. In my experience, this is a major turn-on for ladies — even slightly ahead of hand and foot massage. Move from one toe to the next to the next, spending time to stick your tongue between her toes and lick her "toe crotches." When you get to the baby toe, stick her four small toes into your mouth all at one time and take as much of her foot into your mouth as you can.

  Now: I **always** endeavor to anchor *toe sucking* to *extreme arousal* by reaching up and fingering her vagina (or her clit) while doing this sucking. If her feet are so long (or your arms so short) that you can't reach both her toes and her vulva, bend her leg a bit. Viola.

Lady on her tummy:

- Your head is near hers, your hand between her legs. While employing her favorite fingering techniques, lick and then lightly bite her earlobe — firmly, but not enough to break her state from *feeling* to *thinking*. While biting, you can pull away a bit. Not too hard, pain is not the goal; behaving like an animal is the goal — consider emitting a low growl. The idea, is to associate the ear-play with extreme sexual arousal. If you do this a number of times, you're likely to find that nibbling at her ear will put her into an aroused state immediately. (This is hypnosis 101.) You can also consider simply pinching her earlobe, for that way, you may be able to get her aroused either in public or at the start of your sexual play evening simply by pinching her earlobe.

NOTE: I'm just picking on her earlobe. You may wish to anchor her arousal somewhere else. In one class on sexual hypnosis, I watched the instructor privately anchor this arousal state to a lady's shoulder. About 30 minutes after the anchor was set and everyone was on a snack break, another lady came up to the subject from behind to say something to her. The second she touched that shoulder, the subject's knees buckled, she started shaking with mini-orgasms, and she turned bright red. This drew quite a crowd; the lady who had touched her kept apologizing, saying she had no idea that an anchor was set there. So, you need to use some common sense when picking anchor points, or she might get an orgasm triggered at an inappropriate time or place (grocery store, at her work, in church). Again, this is not some hypothetical point, this comes from my direct experience — and not at the training workshop.

- Same basic activity, but rather than biting or licking her earlobe, make a claw with one hand and firmly claw her body wherever it seems right. Often, clawing the leg works just fine. Again, pain is not the goal; an unusual stimulation is the goal. You're going for *anchoring*.

- You're kneeling next to her with the Oster® massager strapped to the back of your hand. Insert two fingers barely inside the vaginal opening and swirl them around. You're likely to get real sighs of pleasure. Once she's accommodated to this, insert the fingers and curl them around as much of her spongy tissue as you can reach. From here, you can pull up with varying degrees of firmness, depending upon her arousal level. That is, if you're just starting out and this fingering comes after you've oiled her down and provided a nice massage, don't do anything dramatic; keep all the action slow, soft, and dreamy. On the other hand, if you've been playing sexually for an hour or so and want to introduce some variety, this is a way to do so. (Note: Some of these massagers can get pretty hot. Try not to let it touch her thighs. If she's far enough into a trance state and the hot metal touches her skin, you'll break that state. She's likely to jerk and get out of her aroused head-space to ask you what just happened.)

Lady on her knees:

- This technique is better if she's on her knees, but she *can* be on her tummy. Insert two fingers in a downward direction (pointing towards the bed) and stroke her G- and A-spots. In this case, keep your fingers below her cervix. This is one of the easiest ways to reach her A-spot.
- With your thumb in her vagina and your fingers working away in her slit, spank her. Not hard, and not very frequently. Once you are assured that she liked the initial slap, you may then begin to build up to a little — not a lot — more intensity. For some women, the slap adds a tremendous amount of pleasure to all the fingering that you're doing.

A Special Technique Just for Readers

I'd neither heard of nor seen this technique until I met and befriended a fellow from the Netherlands. With a very warmed-up woman on her back, he would gently insert his second and third (and sometimes his fourth) fingers into her, covering most of her vulva with the flat of his hand, palm resting on her mons. He would use fairly vigorous up-and-down fingering motion with one hand, while using his free hand to pound on the back of the inserted hand. Sometimes he would only pound once or twice, at other times, he would pound 6-8 times. This inventive sexual play sent low-vibration shock waves throughout the lady's body. You don't have to pound very hard or very fast. Since you're pounding away on the back of your own hand, you're going to feel more pain than you're dishing out, so this is a self-regulating action.

The number of fingers you can insert, and which fingers you choose to insert are a function of the size of your hand/fingers and your lady's degree of comfort. You certainly don't want to insert an uncomfortable number of digits and then pound your hand. In the first place, she needs to be comfortable before you start this kind of sexual play. In the second place, you run the substantial risk of breaking her state if she has to think about any pain that you're causing.

Going for Screaming Orgasms and/or Female Ejaculation

I can recommend only a few techniques that I have found to be consistently successful in the areas of female orgasms and ejaculation. The first is almost guaranteed to get you a tremendous screaming orgasm — even if she doesn't ejaculate. I mentioned it in the section on vibrator play. It involves the simultaneous use of the Flex-a-Pleaser® and the Hitachi Magic Wand®.

Before you start, be sure she is fully hydrated (lots of water) and that you have ample towels under her. Keep a hand towel handy to dry yourselves off once she's done. While most ladies can be accommodated with only a single fold of a bath towel (two layers), sooner or later, you're going to run into a lady for whom 8 layers of towel may not hold everything.

And don't even *think* about asking her how voluminously she ejaculates. If she has never had that experience, the question, itself, can be mortifying — and very embarrassing. Also, as men tend to be competitive, if she tells you that she usually goes through four towel layers, then you're likely to take that as a challenge, rather than view the entire event as an amazing display of how comfortable she is around you. Also, in this last case, if you can't even get her to ejaculate, you'll now view yourself as being less able than her other lovers. You're not going to want to go there; the question is deadly for each of you.

Safety Warning #11, Repeated: If you're going inside your lady's vagina, wear gloves. If you insist on going in without gloves, then I strongly urge you to trim, buff, and scrub your fingernails before you start. Not to be too extreme about this, you might consider scrubbing fingernails with 90% alcohol (90% because that's about the strongest alcohol on the market) or other hand-sanitizer, and then rinsing them off. You'll become a believer the first time you face the doctor and the medication bills from having given your lady bacterial vaginosis. Unfortunately, this is the voice of experience talking, not some theoretical concept or urban legend.

Tip #29: During most of the sexual play described in this book, I strongly recommend that you spend most of your time reading your lady's facial expressions, breathing rate, and hand gestures. Some ladies suck in their breath and hold it a few seconds just before climaxing; some women display the "sexual flush" at this point (face and/or chest becomes bright red). Also, as she becomes more aroused, note the deepening color of her vaginal lips and listen for changes in her vocalizations. Because you're trying to stair-step your sexual play, these gestures or expressions can be your signal to slow down and back off for a while. Unless she's multi-orgasmic, if you don't back off, you may find that the evening's sexual play has ended.

NOTE: Recall this trick? Depending upon your relationship with your lady, you may want to completely stop the action just short of orgasm and return to appetizers, or pretend you forgot something from the other room and get up and leave. You may even make this an ongoing game between the two of you. Ultimately, the goal of stair-stepping the action is to evoke a substantially stronger orgasm from her than you're likely to get if you go straight from start to orgasm in one single march.

Female Orgasms Using Vibrators

In my experience, one of the surest ways to cause a lady to orgasm from vibrators (as opposed to orgasms created by licking and fingering), involves inserting the Flex-a-Pleaser® vaginally while you're using the Hitachi Magic Wand® or the Wahl 7-in-1® on her vulva. When used together (and with the stimulation stair-stepped), this may well become your most potent combination for producing extremely explosive orgasms.

Remember, we're at Magic Wand® on the outside and Flex-a-Pleaser® on the inside. If you inserted it so that it's pointed downward (woman on her back), you should now rotate it to vibrate over the G-spot. Hold it there. Next, rotate it 180 degrees (back to the downward position) to vibrate over the cervix. Go back and forth between these two orientations. And back and forth and back and forth and... There's plenty of room for improvisation, here, so have a good time. Once you determine whether she is happiest with the inside vibrator vibrating on her cervix or on her spongy tissue (which, by now, has the sensitive

G-spot available in many women) gently rotate the Flex-a-Pleaser® while *slightly* changing the angle and position of the Wand until you can read that you're getting somewhere. At this point, you may want to press a bit harder with the Wand, and also practice slightly twisting the head against her vulva as you increase the pressure. This twisting action will present a new group of sensations to her. Note: For some women, the Wand is too intense to be placed directly on her sensitive skin *between* her outer lips (directly on her clit and the surrounding areas). However, if you *can* do that, this is the time for it.

By this point, your sex partner may begin to howl. Since you're playing the woman like a fine instrument, you may want slightly to change the positions of the two vibrators in order to obtain different volume levels and pitches of howl.

Female Ejaculation Using Your Fingers and Hands

First and foremost, remember that not all women can physically ejaculate. Current research suggests that ejaculate comes from a woman's Skene's glands, and that those glands don't always have openings that exit the body. For this reason, be very, very sure that she is aware of your knowledge of this before you set yourselves up for an unhappy conclusion to your otherwise spectacular sexual evening. Again, this is the voice of personal experience speaking, not some hypothetical concept put in here to protect a woman's feelings.

So, here we go. You've been playing with her for *at* least 30 minutes but, more likely something like 90 minutes or more. She's clearly turned on, and she may be begging for more intense sexual stimulation. With her on her back and you *kneeling* next to her, facing her head, insert two fingers into her vagina and place them firmly over her spongy tissue. For the next five bullets, consider using your index and middle fingers. For the final act, try switching to your second and third fingers, possibly even your fourth. Your purpose, now, is to get her used to more aggressive sexual play.

Please remember:

- Your lady should have taken a trip to the bathroom before you start any of this.
- Your lady should be lying with ample towels underneath her.
- In addition to your lube-of-choice, you will want a hand towel near by.

Spend some initial time stroking her spongy tissue and the inside of her vagina in a variety of ways.

- Use your second and third fingers to capture her spongy tissue and pull it down towards her back.
- Curl your fingers all the way around the spongy tissue to probe for particularly sensitive spots. (Remember, the famous G-spot is not in any particular place on women and can move around on your own lady depending on her level of arousal.)

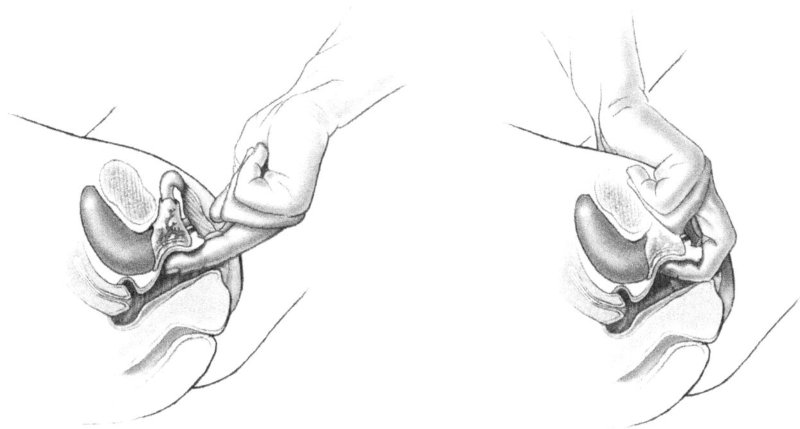

- Perform a wave action with your fingers, going over her spongy tissue.
- Use your fingers to slap her cervix from side to side. This is done by inserting your hand into her vagina in a vertical orientation, fingers together (up and down in line with her slit). Keep your fingers straight out and bent as far back as possible (if you're right handed, then your fingers are bent back to the right). The back side of your fingers should be touching the wall of her vagina. Then, very quickly snap your fingers closed to hit the opposite side of her vaginal wall, brushing her cervix as you go by. Practice with various speeds of opening and closing your hand — see what suits her.

Safety Warning #12: Even if your fingernails were close-trimmed and you scrubbed them clean before your evening began, you must be wearing gloves for this. You risk scratching skin at the end of her delicate cervix if you use your bare hand. As mentioned before, bacteria can be introduced inside your lady from even the most mild insertion of your unclean fingers.

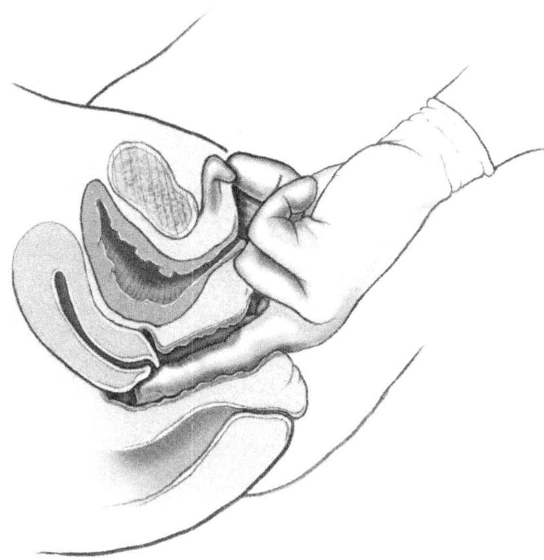

- Once you master the previous technique, rotate your hand so it's palm up and repeat the same action, but now start under her cervix, and end up with your fingers curled around her spongy tissue. If you haven't felt it already, her vagina will now be swollen quite a bit with her advanced arousal. This will feel something like playing around inside a rubber ball that has a protrusion (cervix) in it; lots of open air. (Remember: Not only do women who have had hysterectomies not have a cervix, but the location of the cervix varies somewhat between women. Also, as the vaginal canal elongates with arousal, you may or may not even be able to hit her cervix when your fingers are pointing upward. It depends.)

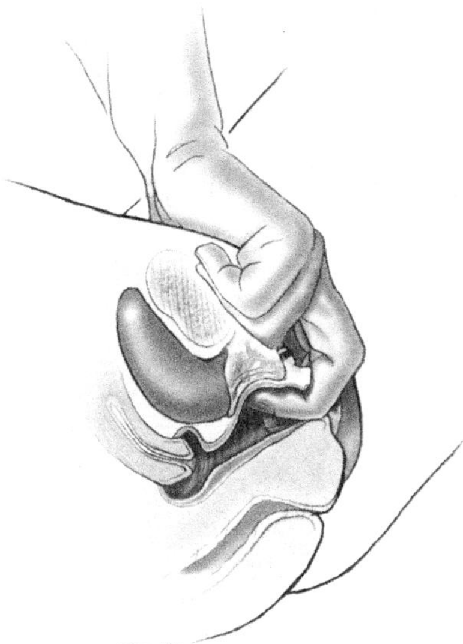

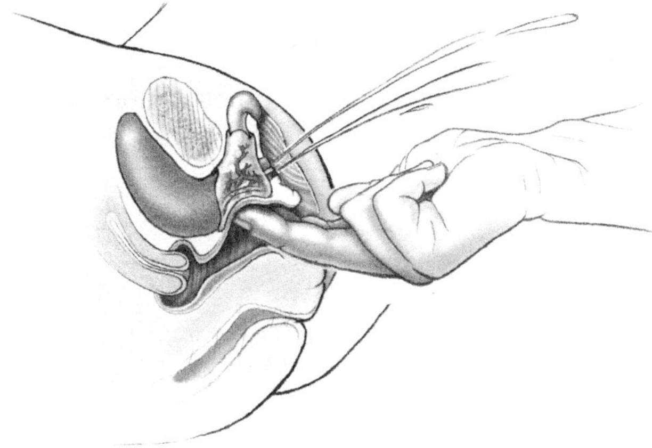

We're coming up to ejaculation. Once she's accommodated to all this vaginal play, you will want to curl your fingers around her spongy tissue and start to pull up and release, rapidly and vigorously (illustration on left). Warning: Some ladies don't go for this. You should have figured this out when you practiced some of the sexual activities we've just been describing. At this point, I'll assume your lady does like this kind of sexual play — which, in my experience, is more the rule than the exception — and I'll continue with the details. (If the "pulling up" action is too intense, you can try positioning yourself as illustrated on the right.)

You need to realize that when you're pulling up, you're not only using your biceps, you're actually (slowly) adding body weight as she gets used to the motion. It's rather like rowing or chopping a tree; you're putting your back into this action, not just your arms. Frankly, unless you're in seriously great physical shape, you'd probably become exhausted if you tried to use only your arms.

Your action, at this point, is largely up to you, but the components to keep in mind are these:

- You're pulling up on her rapidly and fairly vigorously.
- You can alternate this action by quickly switching from a "fingers up" to a "fingers down" position. And back and forth and back...

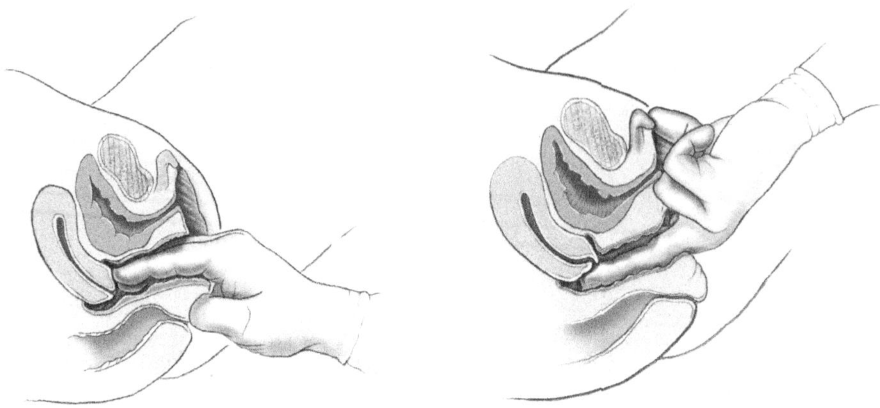

- You can alternate between a "fingers curled around her spongy tissue" position to an open-hand position. As you repeatedly and quickly alternate between these two positions, you should be able to bat her cervix around. Often, this is highly arousing.
- With fingers curled around her spongy tissue, you can extend your fingers about half way between the end of her spongy tissue up to the beginning of her cervix (the A-spot) and massage that area firmly. You'll know you've got it by reading her reactions.
- You can cool the action down a degree by hitting on the back of the hand that is inserted inside her. Not much, just one or two hits; then resume the vigorous up and down action that is the basis of this group of comments. If she's highly vocal, this change in action should produce a really delightful series of sounds.
- You can make up some of your own techniques that are adapted either to your own style of sexual play or to the preferences of your lady.

You're likely to find that this phase goes pretty quickly, perhaps only a few minutes. You will have no problem feeling her ejaculate. As you and your lady do this more and more frequently, my experience has been that the volume of ejaculate increases — sometimes quite dramatically. Over the course of a year, she may go from needing only two folds of towels beneath her to needing eight or more folds of towel to catch all the ejaculate. In rare cases, you may find a woman whose ejaculate is measured more by the cup than by the number of towel folds. If this happens, you may want to put plastic protection under the towels to keep from soaking your bed or other play surfaces. By the way, if you run into a lady like this, she probably knows all about ejaculating and will warn you ahead of time.

After she has ejaculated, slow down your pace so she can recover. As many women can ejaculate a number of times in a row, you may not want to bring her all the way down, right now. If you want to see whether your lady is in that group, ask her permission to begin again to work up to another round of ejaculation. For each of your ladies, you'll need to figure out when and where to start over. I will say, though, that you may want to pat her dry, reapply some lube, and then go back to some licking and vibrating. As she's very aroused at this point, you may wish to suck her clit into your mouth while stroking her spongy tissue with one finger. You're back to slow buildup again. When you determine that she's ready, switch to a kneeling position (facing her) and have at it.

Generally, consider stringing three or four female ejaculation episodes together in an evening. Sometimes a few more; sometimes a few less. As ever, it depends upon the lady and your reading of her level of interest. Often, though, I think you'll find ladies who will urge you on and on and on. Pretty soon, either you'll be too worn out to continue, or she'll be out of fluid.

Fisting — A Brief Note

There may be some times that you might consider following your previous sexual activities with vaginal fisting (having all of your hand inside your lady's vagina). That said, it can easily take you months or years of on-again-off-again work with a lady before you'll be able to get all the way in.

Some women enjoy vaginal fisting, some don't — or don't think that they will and are not inclined to find out. If you're new to this topic, fisting is *definitely* a case where you must proceed only with your partner's active and ongoing encouragement, and within her comfort level. Also, there are many special techniques that you'll need to know. If you two would like to give vaginal fisting a try, then please read Deborah Addington's book A Hand in the Bush: The Fine Art of Vaginal Fisting. If possible, find someone who can give you private instruction. As I said, there are some special techniques involved with fisting, and if you're just doing this from a book, you'll benefit from obtaining help from someone who's done this before.

> **Tip #30:** If you decide to learn how to do vaginal fisting, don't be macho and try to force your way in. Not only will you violate her trust in you and raise questions about her interest in future sexual explorations with you, but you could possibly tear her skin. This is supposed to be a bonding experience, not a project that has to be conquered.

Chapter Summary

This topic is one of my favorites. I opened with some "rules" for early-stage fingering, moved on to a wide range of specific advanced techniques and ended that section by including a very special technique for readers of this book, only. Next, I went over some options you have for bringing your lady to screaming orgasm and possibly to ejaculation. One technique involved a vibrator, the other was exclusively a fingering technique. The chapter closed with a brief tip of the hat about vaginal fisting.

Part V

Epilogue

Chapter Twelve

Winding Down

Bringing Closure to Your Evening

Your sexual evening is likely to be exhausting for you both. While men have a tendency to go to sleep after sex, women who have just gone through the kind of activities described in this book will need some tender aftercare; she'll need time to reconnect with the world. This will be true whether your evening was structured to transition from female ejaculation and orgasm to sexual intercourse, or whether your evening was designed to end before intercourse.

As the guy, you want to avoid simply separating from her and turning on the television. You may be done, but she hasn't landed, yet. The TV noise may not only annoy her, it may make her angry with you. You're likely to have your own idea about how to bring your lady down softly, but if you don't, here are some ideas past the "cradle her in your arms" approach.

- Quietly switch the music to something soft and romantic — without a driving beat
- Bring her a glass of water (don't ask her, just do it)
- Bring a piece of chocolate with the water
- Let her lie still while you rub her back (with or without massage oil)

- Massage her hands and feet
- Stroke her with a feather

You might want to plan for a twenty-minute period while she is readjusting to her environment. During this time, you're trying to avoid bringing her back into her head. That is, you want her to remain in a *feeling state* not in a *thinking state.* Thus, don't ask any questions that engage her brain.

Once she starts to come around, you might consider offering to read her a short story while she remains resting with her head either on your shoulder or in your lap. This is a time of intimate bonding. I'll leave it to you to work out how that will work in your world.

The Next Day

Because you don't want your lady to break her soft and loving mood during your evening together, I suggest that you wait until the next day to get a critique. If you've thought of some questions you'd like to ask her, you may wish to capture them on paper so you can ask her in the morning. Also, if you make some notes about the evening's adventure, you're likely to be better able to create an even more magical evening the next time the two of you are together. A word of caution concerning this discussion. You need to explain to your lady that you are seeking the advice in order to improve her pleasure. You also need to explain that all comments will be welcomed. Now, guys, here's the hard part. If she says something negative, you have to remain neutral. If you go defensive, she'll probably not share with you again. Your task is only to listen attentively and to take notes.

Getting on My Soapbox

Give me a sec while I climb up on my soap-box.

> **Tip #31:** In the words of the John Prine song, I suggest that you "*Blow up the TV.*" Watching television night after night is wasting your life and it detracts tremendously from spending quality time with your partner. I know; it's none of my business. All I can say is that if you use your time reading interesting books (dare I say sex books?) and playing with your lady, not only will you become a more interesting person, but I'd bet money that your relationship will transform into the sexual fantasy life you each had in mind when you first came together.

Okay, that's over. Well, sort-of over...

As I've mentioned throughout this book, I firmly believe that the quality of your sex life will improve dramatically if you adopt an attitude of wonder and amazement that this Woman will give you the unbelievable honor of allowing you to touch her without restrictions. This is true whether applied to the first time you've been with a lady or the three-thousandth time you've been with your partner. I urge you to revel in your good fortune, and to delight in all the curves that are being offered to you. I propose that to the extent that you can make this philosophy your own, your ability to please a woman will increase dramatically.

Closing Statement

I hope you've enjoyed reading this book as much as I have enjoyed writing it. This has given me a chance to share sex techniques that have taken me years to develop — both from substantial research and from personal experience.

As I also said at the beginning, your sex play will probably be improved by changing your view of a sexual encounter, by increasing your range of techniques and skills, and by being able to perform certain acts with consistency.

Final Tip: When you're using the techniques explained in this book, I strongly, strongly urge you to play music that supports this kind of sexual play. To me, that means music where the beats are somewhat different from track to track. Such music is critical to this kind of play, because you will find a number of advantages to using these fingering techniques in time with the music's beat. Not only will this keep you from going too fast and causing her to climax too soon, you will also want to use the 10-20 seconds between tracks to stop your movements entirely. At those interludes, you probably want to remove your fingers from the lady, better to offset your different techniques, but — more importantly — to have an external way to remind yourself that these techniques rely on stair-stepping your action.

I sincerely hope that you will find the information that I have shared with you to be both interesting and useful; I certainly hope that it helps you with your own relationship(s) with Ladies. If you have any questions, please do not hesitate to contact me.

Robert J. Rubel
Bob.Rubel@Yahoo.com

Appendix A

Resources

Book Resources Directly Related to Topics in This Book

Core Readings

Blue, Violet. The Ultimate Guide to Cunnilingus. San Francisco: Cleis, 2002.

This book is obtainable through Good Vibrations at http://www.goodvibes.com. It has lots of very specific techniques. I recommend it highly. Also, it is the only book I ever found that contains a discussion of sexual pressure points. Touching these specific places augments your sex play. I also highly recommend her companion book: The Ultimate Guide to Fellatio.

Chalker, Rebecca. The Clitoral Truth: The Secret World at your Fingertips. New York: Seven Stories, 2000.

This book is the final word about female genital anatomy and what to do with it.

Dawn, Crystal and Stephen Flowers. Carnal Alchemy: a Sado-Magical Exploration of Pleasure, Pain and Self-Transformation. Smithville, Texas: Runa-Raven Press, 2001.

This is a very concise "meaty" book about sex magic. It provides the best descriptions of sex magic (what it is and how to produce it) that I have ever found. This topic is *extremely* hard to research, and the knowledge not easily discovered. Your website reference is: http://www.runaraven.com.

Goddard, Jamie and Kurt Brungart. Lesbian Sex Secrets for Men. New York: Plume, 2000.

Extremely helpful book full of lots of really valuable tips. This is where I learned to love armpits.

Michaels, Marcy. The Lowdown on Going Down: How to Give Her Mind-Blowing Oral Sex. New York: Broadway, 2005.

Written by a PhD speech pathologist, this is the best book I have ever seen about tongue and head exercises and extreme details about what works and why. I recommend it highly.

Stubbs, Kenneth Ray. Kama Sutra of Erotic Massage — The Tantric Art of Touch. Tucson: Secret Garden, 2002.

While you can probably figure out what direction to massage your lady and where to do the massage, this book gives you a good, competent, detailed description. (www.secretgardenpublishing.com)

Venning, Rachel and Claire Cavanah. 101 Sex Toys: a Playfully Uninhibited Guide. New York: Fireside, 2003.

These women are the founders of Toys in Babeland (www.toysinbabeland.com). Excellent orientation to the vast majority of sex toys available to you and their website carries most of them. [Side note: this is one of a very few sex toy shops owned and run by women. It's in Seattle.]

Wiseman, Jay. Tricks... To Please a Woman and its companion, Tricks... To Please a Man San Francisco: Greenery, 2004.

I recommend both books highly; there is very clever stuff in here. He collected sex ideas from people nationwide.

Other Highly Recommended Books

Barker, Tara. The Woman's Book of Orgasm. New York: Citadel, 1997.

Chang, Jolan. The Tao of Love and Sex: The Ancient Chinese Way to Ecstasy. New York: Dutton, 1977.

Easton, Dossie and Janet W. Hardy. Radical Ectasy. Oakland: Greenery, 2004.

Keesling, Barbara. Sexual Pleasure: Reaching New Heights of Sexual Arousal and Pleasure. Alameda: Hunter House, 2005.

I liked this one; it had some good ideas and tips and is congruent with my attitudes about sexual play.

Keesling, Barbara. How to Make Love All Night (and Drive a Woman Wild). New York: Harper Collins, 1994.

Paget, Lou. The Great Lover Playbook: 365 Sexual Tips and Techniques to Keep the Fires Burning All Year Long. New York: Gotham, 2005.

Actually, he's written a number of books that I recommend to you: How to Be a Great Lover, How to Give Her Absolute Pleasure, Orgasms: How to Have Them, Give Them, and Keep Them Coming, and Hot Mamas. I have read most of these.

Winks, Cathy. The Good Vibrations Guide: The G-spot. San Francisco: Down There, 1998.

For men still engaging in intercourse: If you're *really* committed to mastering unending male intercourse, pick up a copy of Ancient Lovemaking Secrets: The Journey Toward Immortality by James W. McNeil (self published: www.littlenineheaven.com or www.sexforhealth.net).

He teaches you how to separate male orgasm from ejaculation so that you can have multiple orgasms yet not ejaculate until you want to. You can attend his workshops in California, or hire him to come to you. He's in his 60s and spent most of his life in the Orient studying sexual ecstasy. I've seen him in action at a national swingers' convention where he had a substantial line of quite-young ladies standing around waiting for him to finish so they could play with him. I was impressed, to say the least. Very interesting fellow. In his book, he's included a photo showing him standing on the peak of his roof, swinging a woman (who is a few feet off the ground) from his genitals. (Hanging weights from your scrotum while repeatedly pinching your buttocks together is a core exercise.)

Books in Specific Areas of Interest

Anal Oral Contact — Analingus

The best website I've seen on this subject is by Violet Blue: http://www.tinynibbles.com/rimshot.html

Two books from my library are very good:

- Morin, Jack. Anal Pleasure and Health: A guide for men and women, second edition. San Francisco: Yes, 1986.
- Taormino, Tristan. The Ultimate Guide to Anal Sex for Women. San Francisco: Cleis, 1997.

Bondage

Wiseman, Jay. Jay Wiseman's Erotic Bondage Handbook. San Francisco: Greenery, 2000.

> Jay is a good friend of mine and if you're interested in starting out with some bondage play, this is absolutely your best first book. (www.greenerypress.com)

Fantasy Sex

Blue, Violet. The Ultimate Guide to Sexual Fantasy: How to Turn Your Fantasies into Reality. San Francisco: Cleis, 2004.

> This is a great book that covers topics such as *public sex, multi-person sex, how to build a fantasy scenario, role play, strip clubs,* and *fetishes,* among other topics. Highly recommended, if you wish to explore a more daring path.

Califia, Patrick. Sensuous Magic: A Guide to S/M for Adventurous Couples. San Francisco: Cleis, 2001.

> Unless you are already a kinkster, I urge you to read Jay Wiseman's SM-101 before you try this one. This one assumes that you know a few things about the world of kinky sex.

Intercourse

If, in fact, you're interested in resources for intercourse, here are two of my favorite items.

Editors of Cosmopolitan Magazine. The Cosmo Kama Sutra: 77 Mind-blowing Sex Positions. New York: Hearst, 2004.

> This is the best sex-position and discussion book I've ever seen.

This web site: http://users.forthnet.gr/ath/nektar/kma/main.htm

This is the best website I've ever seen for sex positions. This site gives you twenty-four animated GIFs. In particular, *The Preludes* closely matches the techniques I'm describing in the section titled: "Female Ejaculation using your Fingers and Hands."

Kinky Sex

Easton, Dossie and Catherine Liszt. When Someone You Love is Kinky. Oakland: Greenery, 2000.

Dossie, a practicing psychologist in the San Francisco area, has co-authored this book to give to a friend or lover to explain to them some of the reasons why you enjoy this lifestyle. The authors take a calm and understanding approach in this book, perfect for non-kinky readers who might wonder why their otherwise "normal-looking" relative takes such delight in activities they, themselves, may be uncomfortable with.

Wiseman, Jay. SM-101: a Realistic Introduction. San Francisco: Greenery, 1996.

This has always been, and remains to this day, the best and most complete introduction to the world of kinky sex. I recommend it very highly. (www.greenerypress.com) See, also: www.jaywiseman.com.

Power Exchange in Sexual Relations

Brame, Gloria, William Brame, and Jon Jacobs. Different Loving: The World of Sexual Dominance & Submission. New York: Villard, 1993.

Again, I urge you to read Jay Wiseman's SM-101 before you try this one. This one is pretty specialized, assumes that you've already started learning about kinky sex, and that you now want to explore *power exchange* in your relationship. In my world, this is a *core reading.*

Power Exchange Books' Reference Series. Las Vegas: Nazca Plains.

This book series discusses power exchange within consensual adult relationships. Each volume features a different type of relationship structure within the world of kink. These books and magazines are available from www.Amazon.com or from http://rubelpresents.com/PEMbooks/.

Spanking

Green, Lady. The Compleat Spanker. Oakland: Greenery, 1996. www.greenerypress.com.

If you even *think* you or your partner gets sexual pleasure out of spanking or being spanked, this is a *must read*. She has a great *resources* appendix.

Music Resources

There is one book on this subject: it is...

Kale, John. Sex Between the Beats: The Ultimate Guide to Sex Music. Venice, California: Blush Books, 2005.

This book comes with a CD that will give you some ideas. I must admit, Kale is preaching the same tune you've run into with this book; carefully selected music will provide a terrific boost to your sexual evening. (www.blushrecords.com)

Beyond the book, here are some specific CDs for you to consider:

- Canyon Trilogy by R. Carlos Nakai (Good "starter" music, as you're just beginning your evening.) Its also good for winding down and aftercare.
- The Secret Door by Mystic Ocean
- Dirty Vegas by Dirty Vegas
- The Best of Delerium by Delerium
- Karma by Delerium

Special Internet Resources

Leather Scented Products

This website is the source-supply for products wholesaled to most of the very large Internet Leather stores: www.leatherstock.com.

Source for a CD of a Thunderstorm

www.f7sound.com/thunder.htm

More Material from Jay Wiseman

www.jaywiseman.com

A Comment Concerning Sexual and/or Emotional Abuse

More women than you might think have had prior experiences with sexual or emotional abuse. I've provided some stats for sexual abuse/rape. For a competent link for information about emotional abuse, see: http://www.WomanAbusePrevention.com/html/emotional_abuse_facts.html).

- Of female Americans who are raped, 54% experience their first rape before age 18. Prevalence, Incidence and Consequences of Violence Against Women: Findings From the National Violence Against Women Survey. Patricia Tjaden and Nancy Thoennes. Washington, DC: National Institute of Justice, US Department of Justice, November 1998.

- Of 18-36 year old females in the US, 57% of Afro-Americans and 67% of white Americans report at least one instance of sexual abuse. "The sexual abuse of Afro-American and white-American women in childhood." G.E. Wyatt. Child Abuse Neglect, Volume 9, number 4, 1985, pages 507-19.

Appendix B

Some Phrases to Transform Your Relationship

These sentences were inspired by the very appropriately-named Mr. Wonderful Doll®, who speaks market-tested phrases that the manufacturer maintains women *really, really* would like to hear from their man. However, you must actually *mean* whatever you choose to say to your mate — otherwise, her BS detector will go off and she'll be furious at you.

- Actually, I *do* seem to be sort-of lost — Let me just pull in here and ask for directions.
- I love you. No, nothing special, I just hadn't told you in a while.
- Yes, Dear, I'll be glad to do that.
- You know, I've been thinking about you all day. That's why I bought you these flowers.
- Love, I'll bet you're tired after your full day; you just rest on the couch and watch some TV while I'll make us dinner tonight. For dessert, I'll rub your feet.
- Hey, the kids are playing at Billy's; how about if I take you down to the mall. I'll bet you can use some new shoes. Then, let's go out for lunch. I really miss spending quality time with you.
- Nah, this ball game really isn't all that important to me; I'd actually rather spend time with you tonight.

- As long as we're cuddled up here on the couch, I don't really care *what* we watch on TV.
- You know, I read that women really need to talk about relationships. How about if we set some time aside this weekend and check in with one another.

About the Author

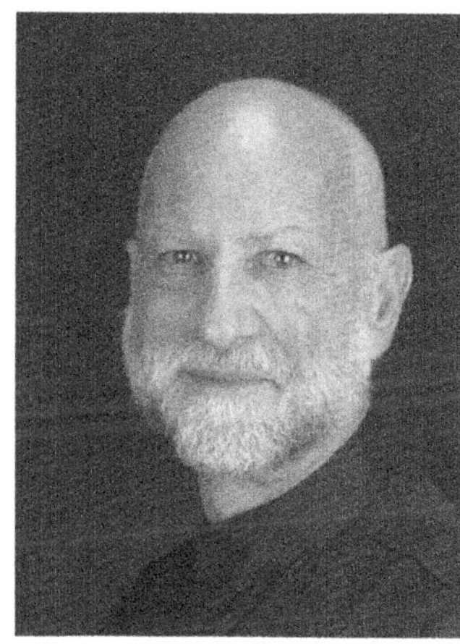

Dr. Rubel is an educational sociologist and researcher by training. Immediately after college he taught high school English in South-Central Los Angeles for three years. Returning to graduate school, he earned an EdM (Boston University) and PhD (University of Wisconsin) in the area of crime prevention in public schools. After serving a stint as a Visiting Fellow at the US Department of Justice, he formed a 501(c)(3) that specialized in crime prevention in public schools. He ran that firm for 17 years. During part of that period, he also was a founding member of the American Association of Woodturners, which he also ran for its first three years of existence.

Robert has extensive management experience with non-profit associations, formerly holding national certification as a Certified Association Executive through the American Society of Association Executives. He is a heavily published author and has served as founder and managing editor of two national quarterlies, one for school police/security directors, and one for his beloved art-form of woodturning. He is an avid dancer, specializing in West Coast Swing and most country-western dance forms.

In his mid-40s, Bob decided to change careers utterly and joined a stock brokerage and future brokerage firm in Washington, DC. Within six months, he was made a Principal of the futures brokerage side of the firm, and five months later was named CEO. He ran the company for the next four years. Upon the request of a close friend, Dr. Rubel returned to Austin to help start a new company. He worked as the corporate operations officer for five years, and then retired to pursue his passion as an erotic and fetish art photographer and writer.

Robert (Bob) Rubel has been involved in the world of alternative sexuality for a number of years, throwing himself into the literature of the field as though it were an academic study. He frequently serves as a presenter at weekend conferences in this field.

Made in the USA
Monee, IL
18 October 2026

66036201R10109